Traumatic Brain Injury Rehabilitation

Services, treatments and outcomes

Edited by

M.A. Chamberlain

Charterhouse Professor of Rehabilitation Medicine
Rheumatology and Rehabilitation Research Unit
Leeds University, UK

V. Neumann

Consultant, Chapel Allerton Hospital, Leeds, UK and
Senior Lecturer in Rehabilitation Medicine
Rheumatology and Rehabilitation Research Unit
Leeds University, UK

A. Tennant

Charterhouse Principal Research Fellow
Rheumatology and Rehabilitation Research Unit
Leeds University, UK

CHAPMAN & HALL MEDICAL
London · Glasgow · Weinheim · New York · Tokyo · Melbourne · Madras

Published by Chapman & Hall, 2–6 Boundary Row, London SE1 8HN, UK

Chapman & Hall, 2–6 Boundary Row, London SE1 8HN, UK

Blackie Academic & Professional, Wester Cleddens Road, Bishopbriggs, Glasgow G64 2NZ, UK

Chapman & Hall GmbH, Pappelallee 3, 69469 Weinheim, Germany

Chapman & Hall USA, 115 Fifth Avenue, New York NY 10003, USA

Chapman & Hall Japan, ITP-Japan, Kyowa Building, 3F, 2-2-1 Hirakawacho, Chiyoda-ku, Tokyo 102, Japan

Chapman & Hall Australia, 102 Dodds Street, South Melbourne, Victoria 3205, Australia

Chapman & Hall India, R. Seshadri, 32 Second Main Road, CIT East, Madras 600 035, India

Distributed in the USA and Canada by Singular Publishing Group Inc., 4284 41st Street, San Diego, California 92105

First edition 1995

© 1995 Chapman & Hall

Typeset in Palatino by Florencetype Ltd., Stoodleigh, Devon.

Printed in Great Britain by Clays Ltd, St. Ives.

ISBN 0 412 48970 8   1 56593 307 9 (USA)

A catalogue record for this book is available from the British Library

Library of Congress Catalog Card Number: 95–69154

Printed on permanent acid-free text paper, manufactured in accordance with ANSI/NISO Z39.48–1992 and ANSI/NISO Z39.48–1984 (Permanence of Paper).

Contents

Contributors

Mike Barnes
Professor of Neurology,
Hunters Moor Rehabilitation
Centre, Newcastle upon Tyne, UK

Eric Bérard
Medical Director,
L'Argentière Medical Centre,
France

Ina J. Berg
University Lecturer,
Department of Neuropsychology
and Gerontology,
University of Groningen,
The Netherlands

Richard Body
Specialist Communication
Therapist, Head Injury
Rehabilitation Centre,
Sheffield, UK

Maggie Campbell
Lead Clinician Physiotherapist,
Head Injury Rehabilitation
Centre, Sheffield, UK

M. Anne Chamberlain
Charterhouse Professor of
Rehabilitation Medicine,
University of Leeds, Leeds, UK

Alex Chantraine
Professor of Physical Medicine
and Rehabilitation, Geneva
Medical School, Geneva,
Switzerland

Anne-Lise Christensen
Professor of Neuropsychological
Rehabilitation, Centre for
Rehabilitation of Brain Injury,
University of Copenhagen,
Copenhagen, Denmark

Janet Cockburn
Senior Research Fellow and
Neuropsychologist, Department
of Psychology, University of
Reading, UK

Betto G. Deelman
Professor of Gerontology,
Department of Neuropsychology
and Gerontology, University of
Groningen, The Netherlands

Chris Evans
Consultant in Rehabilitation
Medicine, City Hospital, Truro,
Cornwall, UK

Luciano Fasotti
Neuropsychologist, Institute for
Rehabilitation Research,
Hoensbroek,
The Netherlands

Ann Goodman-Smith
Director, Brain Injury Services,
Partnerships in Care Ltd,
Northampton, UK

Zeev Groswasser
Professor and Chairman,
Department for Brain Injury
Rehabilitation, Tel-Aviv
University, Ra'anana, Israel

Sandra Horn
Lecturer in Health Psychology,
University of Southampton, UK

David Hughes
Manager in Disability Services,
Leeds City Council, Department
of Social Services, Leeds, UK

Ruth Hunter
Community Occupational
Therapist, Leeds City Council,
Department of Social Services,
Leeds, UK

Marthe Koning-Haanstra
Clinical Neuropsychologist,
Department of Neuropsychology
and Gerontology, University of
Groningen, The Netherlands

Feri Kovács
Neuropsychologist, Institute for
Rehabilitation Research,
Hoensbroek,
The Netherlands

Lindsay McLellan
Europe Professor of
Rehabilitation, University of
Southampton, UK

Vera C. Neumann
Consultant and Senior Lecturer in
Rehabilitation, University of
Leeds, Leeds, UK

Michael Oddy
Director of Head Injury
Rehabilitation Unit,
Ticehurst House Hospital
Wadhurst, UK

Miroslav Palát
Associate Professor, Head of
Department of Rehabilitation
Medicine, Industrial Health
Centre, Bratislava,
Slovakia

Miroslav Palát Jr
Assistant Physician, Institute for
Holistic Medicine, Bernried
Starnberger See, Germany

Debora Prichard
Psychologist, L'Argentière
Medical Centre, Aveize,
France

Agnes Shiel
Research Fellow, Rehabilitation
Research Unit, University of
Southampton, Southampton, UK

Thomas W. Teasdale
Psychologist, Centre for
Rehabilitation of Brain Injury,
University of Copenhagen,
Denmark

Alan Tennant
Charterhouse Principal Research
Fellow, University of Leeds,
Leeds, UK

Elizabeth Ward
Principal Occupational
Therapist, Leeds City Council
Department of Social Services,
Leeds, UK

Heather Warnock
Occupational Therapist, Leeds
City Council, Department of
Social Services, Leeds, UK

Martin Watson
Lecturer in Physiotherapy,
University of East Anglia, UK

Barbara Wilson
Senior Scientist (Special
Appointment), MRC Applied
Psychology Unit, Cambridge, UK

Jacqueline Wood
Chief Speech and Language
Therapist, Royal Hospital and
Home, Putney, London, UK

Foreword

In 1986 the Trustees of the Nuffield Provincial Hospitals Trust decided to develop a major core programme of studies concerned with the organization, development and improvement of services for physically disabled and frail elderly people. This programme developed rapidly due to the enthusiastic response of those in the field; and by 1992 the total value of the programme was in excess of £2 million and currently totals over £3.2 million. It comprised a cohesive matrix of grants commissioned throughout the United Kingdom for work in identified areas which, taken in conjunction with existing grants, formed a comprehensive programme of much-needed studies and research in this field. The whole was to be underpinned by a major study planned and financed by the Trust but conducted by the Royal College of Physicians to survey the existing services being provided by some 180 health authorities. This study, together with concern for the handicapped school leaver, information about the availability of disability services and the care of mild/moderate head-injured persons, formed the prime initial thrust of the programme.

In the case of head injury, the Trust was particularly concerned that there was discontinuity of care for many patients and little evidence as to which treatments were effective. Once patients had stabilized in hospital they were discharged into the community under the care of their general practitioner often without a continuing responsibility from the hospital. The general practitioner was frequently inexperienced and in many districts services for assistance and rehabilitation were rudimentary, fragmented and poorly coordinated. These patients were frequently suffering not just from physical disabilities – in themselves often devastating to a fit young person – but also from personality changes that affected family relationships and the ability to return to work. These strains were compounded by financial difficulties if the patient was the main source of the family income and was unable to obtain compensation for the injury.

The Trust further decided that when the programme was well under way a series of "theme conferences" should be held as a way of disseminating information and raising the level of debate about certain specific areas of research into disability. It was envisaged that these would involve both the Trust's grantholders and those supported by other agencies giving an account of their work to an invited audience consisting of researchers in other related fields, those with a direct service interest and the voluntary sector. It was decided that one such conference should be on the care of the head-injured. Professor Chamberlain was invited to organize this: happily she readily agreed, and with the help of her colleague, Mr Alan Tennant, the conference was held in September 1991 at Leeds University.

All those who attended agreed that the conference itself was an enormous success, due not only to the excellent organization and format of proceedings but also to that exciting amalgam of topics, speakers and delegates that occasionally gels into a scintillating and successful meeting. At one level this resulted in contacts and friendships being established and maintained – and this was reinforced by a very successful newsletter which was started by Mr Tennant following many requests from delegates to be kept in touch with workers and developments in the various countries represented. This success, however, has now been encapsulated in the present volume, which is a compendium of the thoughts, experiences and expertise demonstrated at the meeting and which lifts the original rather simplistic aims and hopes of the Trust to a higher level of understanding of the role and effectiveness of clinical care, case management and multidisciplinary working.

As Professor Chamberlain concludes, '*In brain injury the clinical objective is simple though the problem is inordinately complex. We progress by the sharing of ideas and the continued questioning of existing methods – and we strive to improve the lives of those who have sustained traumatic brain injury.*' The conference and all that has followed has undoubtedly made a significant contribution to that end.

Dr Michael Ashley-Miller
Nuffield Provincial Hospitals Trust
December 1994

Preface

This book is written for all those who seek to improve the lives of those who have sustained moderate or severe head injuries, their families and those who care for them. It is written not only for doctors and therapists, but for planners, managers and members of voluntary and public organizations who are concerned with traumatic brain injury. Those with mild head injuries are many and will need some advice (and certainly some awareness) on the part of those who work and live with them. Those with the most severe head injuries also need to be able to live their remaining days with dignity. However, we have concentrated on what is required for those who have sustained an injury severe enough to lead to acute hospital admission and possibly to a shorter or longer period of rehabilitation.

The book arises from a conference (held in Leeds in 1991), which was supported by the Nuffield Provincial Hospitals Trust. We brought together people who were interested in the rehabilitation of traumatic brain injury from across Europe. We particularly sought those who were responsible for new approaches to treatments, evaluations and service delivery. The resulting book is designed to provide ideas, stimulation and models for those who seek to contribute to better services.

As our audience is diverse we have structured the book in three parts in a way which will allow picking and choosing. The first gives the reader some idea of the size and nature of the problem, both in clinical and epidemiological terms. We hope the size of the problem challenges but does not daunt the reader. Both developed and less developed countries, and communities throughout the world, are faced with the problem of managing TBI and we have therefore provided a range of chapters concerned with experience at national, regional and local levels in both urban and rural communities, in richer and poorer countries. We have encountered few examples of services being started in purpose-built buildings and we have assumed that most of our readers will have to develop new services alongside or out of established ones.

The second part of the book is concerned with treatment. Instead of providing a comprehensive review of all aspects of treatment, we have chosen to present the reader with some distinctive approaches and innovations in treatment. Some of these approaches are controversial. Others are widely accepted. We hope that the reader faced with an individual with severe brain injury unresponsive to current management will use them when considering what further different approaches may be tried.

Some readers will be familiar with some treatments at considerable depth. Others will not. We have tried to pursue a middle course, but other texts may have to be consulted if further details are required.

The final section deals with evaluation. Across the world there is a call to provide evidence for the effectiveness of services. This presents particular difficulties for rehabilitation: being a new specialty, its value tends to be underestimated by others. Furthermore, measuring the outcome of rehabilitation is notoriously difficult. Unfortunately, the tendency is to measure what can most easily be measured; providing resources on this basis is all too prevalent. The final section of the book represents an attempt to redress this fault. In it, there are examples of many individual approaches to outcome measurement. We trust this section will enable both those who treat or care for brain-injured people and those who plan services for them to examine the efficacy of different interventions.

If this book encourages its readers to explore new approaches to service design and treatment and encourages a scientific and critical appraisal of these approaches, it will have succeeded in its aim.

M. Anne Chamberlain
Vera C. Neumann
Alan Tennant
Leeds, February 1995

Acknowledgements

We would wish to thank the Nuffield Provincial Hospitals Trust for sponsoring the meeting which gave rise to this book. We would also wish to thank our secretaries, Jackie Packter and Betty Glossop, and our husbands/wife for their invaluable help and patience. Our deep appreciation goes to Christine Pickles for coordinating and compiling the text.

PART ONE
Aspects of service delivery

Head injury – the challenge:

principles and practice of service organization

1

M. Anne Chamberlain

INTRODUCTION – HOW THE CHALLENGE IS SEEN

Those working with head-injured patients know the nature of the problem which confronts them in their particular sphere. Thus, the casualty surgeon will be aware of the range of problems seen in his department daily, from the infant who has fallen down a few steps and appears unscathed, to the tiler who has fallen off a roof at a time when he was earning a little extra money and was not insured by employers, through to the victim of a horrendous road traffic accident with multiple injuries, and, finally, to the unsteady, elderly person whose fall presages the end of independent existence. It is easy for this doctor to appreciate that factors such as alcohol, poor home design and lighting, perhaps contributed to such accidents. The neurosurgeon's view of head injury may be that of dramatic intervention, often with equally dramatic recovery but sometimes with persistent coma or persistent vegetative state. He will also be aware of Jennett's [1] observation that hypoxia and hypotension, and consequent increased disability, may result from delay in reaching the neurosurgical unit.

It is not easy for the neurosurgeon or trauma specialist to acquire a knowledge of long-term outcomes. Conversely, professionals involved in rehabilitation will have a view based almost entirely on that range of cases which they treat at a later stage. The carer has an intensive and protracted understanding of his particular injured relative. Finally, the patient himself will have a view based on his individual range of impairments and his insight into these.

For a service to be effective, the insights of each group of professionals involved, and of patients and carers, and those which arise from the epidemiological considerations outlined in the following chapter, must be incorporated in an overview. Only by being aware of the nature and scope of the problems and the potentials for change can we begin to lay down a strategy that will lead to effective service provision. Thus, part of the challenge still remains that of assembling the proper information, recognizing the need for an adequate response to the problems uncovered.

The Oxford English Dictionary defines a challenge as 'a calling to account' or 'exception is taken' or 'a summons to a trial, contest, game or duel'. We will take this third definition – the summons to a contest – as our working definition of a challenge and realize too that we may well be called eventually to another challenge – have we produced change? The contest with head injury and its sequelae is that of widening the injured individual's narrowed horizons and improving his quality of life and that of his family.

THE CHALLENGES

THE FIRST CHALLENGE: THE FREQUENCY OF BRAIN INJURY

The duel was, until recently, a contest with a shadowy figure. Head injury has been described as 'a silent epidemic'. Head injury is at least 35 times as common as spinal cord injury and yet the services for it are underdeveloped in virtually every country in the world. The reasons for this may be related to the fact that a great deal of head injury has come about relatively recently with increasing motorization of transport, itself a feature of the late 20th century. The developed countries are here probably only a few years ahead of their less developed neighbours, for even where economies are poor there are huge pressures from within society for access to the freedom and status that a car brings. The public seems inured to traffic accidents and fails to recognize the consequent profound disability which is not visible.

The development of a service may depend on medical leadership. Spinal injury services in the United Kingdom are the result of the vision of one man, Ludovic Guttman, developed at a time when one man's vision was extremely influential in the health services. Now it is likely that many in management, as well as medicine, need to be persuaded of the need for change before change can occur.

CHALLENGE TWO: THE LENGTH OF SURVIVAL

As we shall see in the next chapter, the incidence of head injury is high, with one person being admitted to hospital every 6 minutes in the UK. However, it is not this feature itself which is the prime cause of the great challenge. It is the length of survival of those with severe injury – 50 years on average. Most patients who have had a head injury will return to normal living (Chapter 3), but each year a significant number of severely disabled survivors enter the total pool – survivors with very considerable needs who may well require the family or society to put in a great deal of care over a long time with little improvement, and indeed eventually with deterioration, over this time. The needs of those in persistent coma and the cost of providing for these needs also has to be borne in mind, even though these needs are not the thrust of this chapter.

CHALLENGE THREE: THE YOUTH OF VICTIMS

The youth of victims (most are 18–25 year-olds), their lost potential (most of them are at the beginning of their wage-earning capacity) and the length of time they will have to endure the disabilities subsequent on injury result in the high prevalence of disability referred to above. These factors and the fact that the long process of growth to a fully responsible adult is disrupted lead to frustration and anxiety. The youth of the patients also requires that professionals be responsive as to their changing needs over time.

CHALLENGE FOUR: THE BURDEN OF DISABILITY

It is not easy to find figures that will help one to quantify the costs of disability. The general statement that disability is never cheaper than normality holds good. The individual's costs will be for such things as care, the relief of carers, the increased wear and tear on equipment and clothing that follow the use of a wheelchair, the use of medication and, in some countries, the cost of seeking medical care. The costs to the disabled individual include the loss of employment; these costs extend to the carers in many instances. (There is the corresponding loss of taxes to the state.) In some cases there are the costs of residential, institutional care; in others the costs of adapting the home, or possibly buying one that is more suitable.

There are also costs to society: the cost to the National Health Service of the UK has been estimated by Wade [2], when discussing services for patients with head injury, as some £100 000 per case of moderate or severe disability in their first year and possibly £500 000 or more during their lifetime. If that patient were to get a contracture, at least a further £10 000 could be added. Pressure sores also increase costs dramatically. Occupational therapy, social work, day centre and various home-based support services might have to be provided by social services. In addition, there might be costs to the education department for younger persons who had sustained brain injury and needed extra help at school.

If a patient required treatment not available on the Health Service in the UK, those costs would increase dramatically; a figure of some £1400 per week for 2 years is not uncommon.

Even this very elementary discussion shows that the burden of doing nothing, or doing something badly and without proper coordination, is likely to be large. This should be a powerful argument for change.

CHALLENGE FIVE: THE VARIETY OF HANDICAPS

Traumatic brain injury is associated with some characteristic patterns of impairment. These not only encompass a huge range of physical, cognitive and emotional problems, but also interact with each other and with environmental factors and premorbid social problems such as alcohol abuse, unemployment, poor attainment at school and poor housing. As a result, the ultimate handicap is unpredictable.

It would be easier to plan for individual patients if we could prognosticate easily, yet even after apparently prolonged unconsciousness some patients recover. Nevertheless, the findings of Evans [3] hold good overall – that unconsciousness for longer than 3 weeks will rarely allow a person to achieve an independent existence. The length of post-traumatic amnesia gives us some indication of outcome, as indeed does the Glasgow Coma Scale [4,5], which predicts survival. However, we need predictions that relate more precisely to the disability that is likely to ensue in the particular individual so that remediation may be most effectively focused. Thus Shiel and Horn's work is of great significance (Chapter 19). In this area, prediction of recovery, the ability to prevent secondary disabilities, avoidance of further impairment and any potential for early treatment to reduce disability are potentially of major importance. Even in developed countries, resources for health are scarce and, for rehabilitation of complex disability, very scarce. Anything we can do in the field of screening, prognostication and audit to reduce inappropriate use of resources, release them for better use and focus such resources as we have is of value. Research here is of the greatest importance.

The severity of the deficits relates closely to the burden of disability. It is this summation of a variety of problems, which are in many areas and which are often numerous or all of great severity, which makes the burden for the patient and family so large in the severe and moderate cases. Unlike a purely physical disability, the patient has lost some of the very skills which would help him adapt to a new situation. Grosswasser [6] and colleagues have shown that the old assumption that head-injured children do better than head-injured adults is not true. Indeed, contrary to traditional thinking, severely injured children learn no faster than comparably injured adults, i.e. slower than their peers: the gaps in learnt material enlarge over time.

However, it is important not to take a nihilistic approach that would potentially deny services to those who can often benefit. Eames and Wood [7] discuss the methods of producing improvement in function, even late after injury. Christiansen (see Chapter 8) and her co-workers, treating their patients in blocks of several months (in University terms), produced measurable improvements. Oddy [8] showed that even 7 years after injury improvement can occur in response to structured therapy. Although the learning process is disturbed in most patients, some potential for learning remains and must be harnessed. However, when planning services, it is important to remember that the patient may not be able to generalize from a particular situation and that learning is probably best accomplished in the real situation or one as close to this as possible. Children with learning difficulties respond similarly, and we should probably learn something from these practitioners and from educational theory in general.

CHALLENGE SIX: THE FAMILY

Too often the family is left on the sidelines during the acute drama of life and death. They do not expect their loved one to survive and when he does they initially equate survival with 'all is well'. However, all is far from well in many cases and the family may have been either ill-prepared for such news or unreceptive to it. In many parts of the world there will be nothing more than this acute phase. Thereafter the family is left to cope with a problem they do not understand and they cannot solve. The challenge here is to use the goodwill and capabilities of the family to best effect, something that is rarely done well.

There is probably an infinity of challenges, but the final one I wish to make is that of interagency working.

CHALLENGE SEVEN: INTERAGENCY WORKING

In more developed countries a variety of agencies, principally health, social services and education, can be called on to help. One could be forgiven for believing that at every interagency boundary there may be interagency disputes, cracks and crevices down which the patient and family may disappear. It is a challenge for us all to negotiate these boundaries well in an arena that is changing fast.

The pattern of working in both health and social fields varies enormously, even across Europe [9]. Thus, the UK is distinguished not only by the strength of its primary care but by the multiplicity of charitable and voluntary agencies that work, mainly in the social sphere, for patients' benefit. The situation is confused at present by the implementation of the Community Care Act, whose philosophy is generally welcomed, with many people agreeing that services should be responsive to those who need them. Nevertheless, many have anxieties about funding and practicalities.

The organization of rehabilitation services differs across Europe and in Eastern Europe it may be concentrated around spas currently suffering greatly from lack of resources. Professor Palát (Chapter 7) describes his unit's successful attempt to bring services from the local hospital to the home.

In some parts of the world services may be highly planned and well funded on a regional basis (e.g. in Sweden). In Australia successful planning has been instigated by insurance for comprehensive rehabilitation in the Sydney area.

In the USA some have access to the highest technology and a level of therapist resourcing unknown in most parts of the world. Yet, many patients have no access to rehabilitation until funding is agreed, and frequently no community follow-up is available. Large sections of the population are uninsured. Finally, while 80% of disabled people live in the developing world, only 10% of the resources to help disabled people are expended there. It is against this background that the next section has to be read.

WHAT FACILITIES AND TREATMENTS DOES THE PATIENT REQUIRE?

The aim of service provision is to minimize residual handicap in all the spheres indicated on the ICIDH [10] classification. These are:

1. orientation;
2. physical independence;
3. mobility;
4. occupation;
5. social integration;
6. economic self-sufficiency.

The family and society require that the burden of disability be reduced, not only in financial but in practical and emotional terms. Resources devoted to head injury must be used to maximum effect. Wherever possible, it is better to build on existing general rehabilitation and support services rather than establish totally new services [2]. We would also expect that an equitable proportion of the gross national product would be devoted to health and social services and that patients would have equality of access, as discussed by Culyer [11]. When planning services, local information will be needed about the numbers and characteristics of those requiring services; in the next chapter we see a considerable variation from area to area.

FEATURES OF A PROPOSED SERVICE

Services for those with head injuries must be comprehensive, coherent, dealing with the patient from the time of accident to his final placement, hopefully at home. In the UK, for every 10 patients who receive financial compensation there are 90 who have no access to finances. This causes much anguish: we should ensure that the infrastructure for all in-patients in all countries is satisfactory.

THE FRAMEWORK OF A SERVICE RESPONSE TO HEAD INJURY

A working party set up in West Yorkshire, UK, in 1988 to consider services for head-injured patients came up with a framework for service provision that has stood the test of time [12]. This is:

- **Phase I: Acute phase**. This extends from the site and time of accident through to the acute hospital episode, possibly with admission, perhaps with neurosurgical intervention. It ends when the patient is discharged or passes to any of the subsequent phases.
- **Phase II: Focused in-patient rehabilitation**. This consists of intensive, focused, multiprofessional team-based in-patient rehabilitation.
- **Phase III: Community-based rehabilitation**. The patient now lives at home, but rehabilitation may take place at home or in Health Authority, Local Authority or voluntary society accommodation. It continues the rehabilitation begun in Phase II. Patients may pass from Phase I to Phase III if they do not need Phase II. Treatment has to be coordinated and based on assessment of changing, multiple needs.
- **Phase IV: Maintenance and support**. Some patients will be unable to return to full activity and work. They and their families may require a regular input which is largely supportive, often for a long period of time. There may be a need for review, or for some intermittent rehabilitation.

In Phase I primary prevention is of importance, including measures designed to improve safety on the roads to decrease both the vulnerability of children, particularly in poor environments, and the effects of high-density, high-speed traffic. Legislation to discourage drinking and driving may be required. It has been suggested that 25% of disability consequent on road traffic accident injuries is preventable. Secondary prevention is of importance. This relates to hypoxia and hypotension, contractures, pressure sores, poor nutrition and other factors (Chapter 9).

While primary prevention, and indeed acute surgical intervention, will vary little from country to country, the services put into place to deal with the needs of patients in Phases II–IV will differ greatly. Thus, in a small cohesive country such as Israel, it is feasible to base all rehabilitation on a single institute (Chapter 3). Similarly, in Denmark, which is small and well resourced, most of the population will find accessible the later educational provision described by Christensen (Chapter 8). This would not be so for an intensely rural, dispersed population. Evans describes the model he uses in Cornwall, UK (Chapter 5) – a central in-patient resource for early head injury and stroke rehabilitation followed by the use of small, local rehabilitation teams conversant with facilities in their own locality. Palát's contribution (Chapter 7) is interesting, for it deals with the balance that has to be struck between providing physiotherapy services centrally (where expensive equipment can be best used) and providing them within the home. Here the patient learns best what he needs to learn; he also expends less energy in accessing the service. However, the physiotherapist travelling across the city will be available to treat few patients, and the resource implications of both methods need careful study. We have to acknowledge, also, that there are no Occupational Therapists in Czechoslovakia (now the new Czech and Slovak Republics), so that the work required of a physiotherapist in treating head injury may differ from what is done in other areas.

CONCLUSION

The contest with head injury is a most difficult one. The battle is unequal for those with severe disabilities, but for a large number of people with moderate or mild disabilities the presence of a properly constructed service may well prove invaluable. If this is well run and bears a close relation to the demographic characteristics of the user group, as well as to the characteristics of the country and health service in which the service is set; and is flexible and innovative, making maximum use of resources that already exist, it is likely that it will produce effects which are to the greater good of patient and carer. It is important that these benefits are quantified so that those who follow afterwards may have the evidence which will help them continue the struggle to enhance facilities for their patients.

REFERENCES

1. Gentleman D, Jennett B. Audit of transfer of unconscious head-injured patients to a Neurosurgical Centre. *Lancet* 1990; **335**: 330–334.
2. Wade DT. Policies on the management of patients with head injury: the experience of the Oxford Region. *Clinical Rehabilitation* 1991; **5**: 141–155.
3. Evans C. Rehabilitation of head injury in a rural community. *Clinical Rehabilitation* 1987; **1**: 133–137.
4. Jennett B, Bond MR. Assessment of outcome after severe brain damage. *Lancet* 1975; **i**: 480–484.
5. Teasdale G, Jennett B. Assessment of coma and impaired consciousness. A practical scale. *Lancet* 1974; **2**: 81–83.
6. Groswasser Z, Costeff H, Tamir A. Survivors of severe traumatic brain injury in childhood. I. Incidence, background and hospital course. *Scandinavian Journal of Rehabilitation Medicine* 1985; **12**(Supp): 6–9.
7. Eames P, Wood RL. Rehabilitation after severe brain injury: a follow-up study of a behaviour modification approach. *Journal of Neurology, Neurosurgery, and Psychiatry* 1985; **48**: 613–619.
8. Oddy M, Coughlan T, Tyerman A, Jenkins D. Social adjustment after closed head injury: a further follow-up seven years after injury. *Journal of Neurology Neurosurgery, and Psychiatry* 1985; **48**: 564–568.
9. Hermanova H. State of rehabilitation medicine in Europe in 1990 and targets for the year 2000. In: *The National Concept of Rehabilitation Medicine*. London: Royal College of Physicians of London, 1991: pp 21–31.
10. World Health Organization. *The International Classification of Impairments, Disabilities and Handicaps*. Geneva: World Health Organization, 1980.
11. Culyer AJ. The promise of a reformed NHS: an economists' angle. *British Medical Journal* 1991; **302**: 1253–1256.
12. Chamberlain MA (Chairman). *The Ideal Management of Head Injury*. Leeds: West Yorkshire Working Party, 1988.

The epidemiology of head injury   2

Alan Tennant

INTRODUCTION

How many people need rehabilitation after a traumatic brain injury (TBI)? It is important to know the scale of the demand for rehabilitation services and an epidemiological perspective can provide this. It requires an examination of a wide range of material. A useful starting point in the UK is the 'Hospitalized Incidence Rate' of head injury. This is the number of new (annual) cases admitted to hospital following a head injury and is usually presented as a rate per 100 000. Most countries that routinely collect data about hospital admissions can provide this statistic, either at the local or regional level. Table 2.1 shows such data for 13 regions or countries reported in the literature over the last decade [1–13] and the rates vary from 152 per 100 000 people in Rhode Island, USA to 468 per 100 000 people in San Marino, Italy.

At first glance these data suggest that the variation between reported incidence rates is limited at most to a magnitude of three. However they mask substantial variation caused by differences in the way in which they are collected and presented.

One of the major contributing factors to this artefactual variation is the desire to differentiate between 'head injury' on the one hand and 'potential' or actual brain injury on the other. This difference is crucial for planning services, as it is the latter that are likely to contribute to the pool of those needing rehabilitation. Considerable debate revolves around which subset of the relevant codes of the International Classification of Diseases, Injuries and Causes of Death (ICD) [14] (which are usually used to classify those admitted to hospital) should be used. Table 2.2 shows the major ICD codes used to compile the Hospitalized Incidence Rate.

Table 2.1 Incidence of admission to hospital for head injury in various regions (rate per 100 000, all ages)

Region/country	Rate
San Marino (Italy)	468
NSW, Australia	392
Ravenna, Italy	372
Denmark	332
Scotland	331
South Africa	316
Aquitaine, France	281
Askershus, Norway	236
Virginia, USA	208
Norway	200
Switzerland	194
San Diego, California	180
Rhode Island, USA	152

Occasionally other codes are used to try to focus on 'actual' brain injury, for example those associated with cranial nerve injuries (870–873; 950–951). Also supplementary information (such as the presence of seizures or vomiting) is sometimes used to qualify codes which 'raise the suspicion of TBI' [6]. Unfortunately this additional information is not always available.

A major contention surrounds 'fracture of the facial bones' (802), which is often excluded on the grounds that it is clearly not brain injury. Others suggest that any injury serious enough to cause this sort of damage is sufficient for inclusion as indicative of potential brain damage. Thus all the figures presented in Table 2.1 use different methods of case

Table 2.2 International Classification of Disease – principal codes used for head injury

Fracture of the skull – 800–804

800	Fracture of the vault of the skull
801	Fracture of the base of the skull
802	Fracture of the face bones
803	Other and unqualified skull fractures
804	Multiple fractures involving skull or face with other bones

Intracranial injury, excluding those with skull fracture – 850–854

850	Concussion
851	Cerebral laceration and contusion
852	Subarachnoid, subdural and extradural haemorrhage, following injury
853	Other and unspecified intracranial haemorrhage, following injury
854	Intracranial injury of other and unspecified nature

ascertainment. For example, the French data exclude fracture of the facial bones, though the South African data would include it if supported by other evidence, for example headaches or vomiting within 5 days. This makes international comparisons of this type very difficult and there is an obvious need to standardize case ascertainment in some way.

Differential methods of case ascertainment are further complicated by the way in which data are presented. Some report rates as 'age-adjusted', for example to the 1960 USA population structure. This means that the overall rate presented is not the rate for that region, but what would be the overall rate if the individual age-specific local rates were applied to, say the 1960 USA population structure. In principle this type of standardization [15] provides a way of comparing different regions or for example different ethnic groups, where their population age structures vary. As age is, as shown below, one of the 'real' causes of variation in incidence rates, differences between regions or ethnic groups may be due solely to their differing age structures, and it is important to take account of this when making comparisons.

There are other concerns, which are rarely mentioned. The most important is the quality of code assignment at the individual hospital level. How reliable are these data at the local level? How well do those inputting data understand the meaning of the coding used and how conscientious are they in seeking to categorize entries correctly? An examination of the assignment to different codes between hospitals can be illuminating. Background work on data presented below on incidence in an English region suggests that variation in the practice of assignment between hospitals could limit the usefulness of the data. For example, only 'intracranial injuries' at the aggregate level (850–854) can be used because some hospitals assign solely to the residual category of 'Intracranial injury of other and unspecified nature' (854), not using the 850–853 codes at all. Thus any attempt to focus on, say codes 851–854, omitting the 'concussion' code 850, would fail in this particular health region because of the crude way in which some hospitals assign codes.

All these concerns about quality, case ascertainment and presentation of data will need to be considered before data are used as a basis for planning services. The crucial point is that the basis for any calculation is clearly understood. However, as Lyle and colleagues argue [2], distinguishing between potential and actual brain injury is important for a service-provider perspective. In their work in New South Wales, Australia, they reduced the incidence from a reported 392–180 per 100 000 after focusing on 'actual' brain injury.

As well as these methodological problems, there is evidence to support the idea that social and demographic factors cause 'real' variation in incidence, and thus affect local service needs. Table 2.3 presents some of the key factors which consistently cause variation in rates.

Table 2.3 Incidence of admission to hospital for head injury in various regions; age, gender, environmental and ethnicity (rate per 100 000).

Type			Region/country	Rate
Age-specific		(0–15)	Scotland	290
		(0–7)	Israel	171
		(0–14)	Cantabria, Spain	139
		(15–19)	Virginia, USA	407
Gender-specific		Males	Aquitaine, France	384
			Askershus, Norway	307
			Minnesota, USA	270
		Females	Aquitaine, France	185
			Askershus, Norway	164
			Minnesota, USA	116
Age-gender specific	♂	10–19	Askershus, Norway	489
	♀	30–39	Askershus, Norway	68
	♂	15–24	Minnesota, USA	658
Environment		Inner city	Chicago, USA	403
Ethnicity (same district)		Blacks	Chicago, USA	394
		Whites	Chicago, USA	196

Age, gender, environment and ethnicity are all shown to be associated with varying incidence of admission to hospital and there are clear indications that interaction between these terms can lead to either very high or very low incidence rates [5,7–9,16–19]. So males show consistently higher rates than females, younger, particularly 'teenage', groups show high incidence and combinations of these characteristics – younger males – give the highest incidence rates. Inner city environments have also been shown to have high incidence rates and, in the same district in the USA, blacks have been shown to have an incidence twice that of their white neighbours. Thus the evidence from these data suggest that there is considerable potential for complex interactions that could elevate or depress incidence rates to a significant degree.

INCIDENCE IN AN ENGLISH REGION

Data from the North West Regional Health Authority (NWRHA) in the UK provides an opportunity to examine some of these factors and to look at 'real' variation in one district. Here much of the artefactual variation that causes problems in comparing findings from different countries can be avoided, because in comparing different districts in one region it is possible to use the same data set and the same case ascertainment codes. The data used include information about every patient discharged from hospital during the year 1986, including demographic details, cause, diagnosis, operations and outcome. Patients were counted as being head-injured if they had one or more condition defined under the ICD codes 800–804 and 850–854. Discharges excluded within- or between-hospital transfers to avoid the problem of double counting. The Region had 19 Health Districts ranging from city areas like Manchester through smaller towns like Wigan and commuter 'satellite' towns like Bury and Blackburn to more rural districts like Lancaster. The region's resident population was just above 4 million in 1986.

Table 2.4 shows the 1986 incidence of head injury for the region, expressed as a rate per 100 000 population.

Table 2.4 Discharges in the North Western Region of the UK, after head injury in 1986, by age and sex of patient (expressed as the rate per 100 000 people in the age–sex group, and in total)

Age group (years)	Sex		Total
	Male	Female	
0–4	999	582	795
5–9	672	343	512
10–14	488	250	373
15–19	612	264	441
20–24	648	244	448
25–29	459	162	313
30–34	276	109	193
35–39	264	142	204
40–44	236	110	174
45–49	197	86	142
50–54	162	72	117
55–59	138	58	97
60–64	116	46	79
65–69	137	59	94
70–74	213	107	151
75–79	382	157	236
80–84	787	188	353
85+	1562	474	711
Total	413	186	297

The overall figure of 297 per 100 000 was consistent with the other reported findings and, as expected, the rate among males was twice that of females. Rates were also high among both the young and the old. These data are presented graphically in Figure 2.1, and the slightly U-shaped incidence curve is typical of hospital admission following head injury in the UK [20].

Table 2.5 shows the data as discharge rates per 100 000 resident population in the various districts that make up the region.

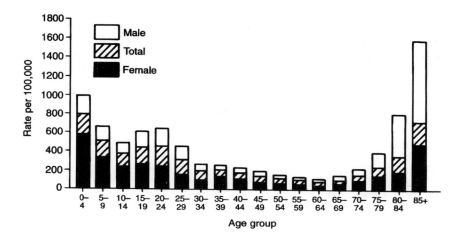

Figure 2.1 Incidence of head injury in an English region.

Rates are shown for males and females, in total and standardized to the region's population. This latter figure gives an indication of the true comparison between districts, having accounted for any variation in age–sex structures of their constituent populations. At the district level discharge rates vary considerably, ranging from 88 per 100 000 residents in Trafford, to 886 per 1000 in Preston, a 10-fold difference. Districts with regional neurosurgical facilities are highlighted. Standardization results in some minor changes but suggests that there are no dramatic differences in the underlying age–sex structures of the different districts.

These rates must be treated with some caution as the denominator used is the resident population, acting as a surrogate for the true denominator, the population at risk. The latter is the average number of people at risk in the district during the year. In other words one must determine, for example, what the average population is, taking into consideration movement for work and leisure. Where there is considerable movement of population, as in Manchester, the task of determining the true at-risk population is substantial, so it is also useful to look at incidence by place of residence rather than discharge. Table 2.6 shows the overall discharge rate amongst residents to be 275 per 100 000 population, a slight fall on the figure given above because it removes those treated in the region who live elsewhere. Once again at the district level rates vary considerably, ranging from 155 per 100 000 in Bolton to 623 per 100 000 in Blackburn, a fourfold difference.

Table 2.5 Discharges after head injury in 1986, by district of discharge and sex of patient (expressed as sex-specific and total rates per 100 000 resident population, together with standardized rates)

District	Sex		All	Standardized
	Male	Female		
Trafford	126	52	88	89
Burnley	226	86	154	152
Bolton	214	100	156	153
Blackpool	202	111	153	169
Salford	236	106	169	176
Wigan	266	133	198	197
Rochdale	302	147	223	215
Tameside	332	176	263	254
Bury	362	156	258	257
Stockport	346	172	256	259
West Lancs	353	176	263	259
Oldham	402	220	309	308
Blackburn	539	247	389	385
South Manchester	594	204	391	396
Central Manchester	698	215	455	442
Lancaster	717	308	502	531
Chorley	752	388	568	557
North Manchester	1083	381	722	735
Preston	1221	571	886	881
Total	414	186	275	–

The fact that the magnitude of difference is different when looking at discharges by district as opposed to district of residence, suggests considerable mobility in the population. Table 2.7 supports this, comparing the two sets of figures on a district-by-district basis.

Those districts with a negative difference export their residents with head injuries to those districts with a positive difference. The three Manchester districts all treat many patients from other districts, as do Chorley, Lancaster and Preston. All are centres of employment in the region. Those districts with large negative differences include many districts to the north of Manchester with large commuting populations. The net balance between the two rates of 22 per 100 000 represents the rate of treatment of out-of-region patients. Clearly an understanding of the complex flows of people between districts is another important factor to be considered in determining demand for rehabilitation services.

From this simple set of data how can we focus down on 'potential brain injury' rather than head injury in general? Given that the underlying code assignments appear to vary between hospitals, we can have little confidence in removing one or more codes. A crude, but perhaps effective alternative for identifying the potential pool of those requiring

Table 2.6 Discharges after head injury in 1986, by district of residence and sex of patient (expressed as sex-specific and total rates per 100 000 resident population, together with standardized rates)

District	Sex		All	Standardized
	Male	Female		
Bolton	220	93	155	152
Trafford	239	90	162	164
Blackpool	222	117	166	182
Salford	249	113	179	185
Wigan	261	125	191	190
Bury	317	137	224	225
Tameside	319	139	226	227
Chorley	307	166	236	241
South Manchester	367	126	242	244
Burnley	362	162	259	256
Stockport	371	172	268	271
Rochdale	418	203	308	297
Lancaster	409	183	290	307
Oldham	466	219	339	339
Central Manchester	516	192	354	342
West Lancs	470	237	352	345
North Manchester	526	195	356	361
Preston	717	354	530	527
Blackburn	857	401	623	615
Total	383	173	275	–

rehabilitation would be to use length of stay as a threshold. In this region 74% of patients are discharged in 2 days or less. While not underestimating the problems caused by minor head injury, a stay of 3 days or more may provide a better indication of likely demand for rehabilitation.

Sex-specific incidence for discharge after head injury requiring at least 3 days in hospital is shown in Table 2.8.

The figures are presented as discharges from districts and show nearly an 11-fold difference in incidence. Differences emerge in the proportion of patients who stay for longer than 3 days. Blackburn, which consistently showed high rates of discharge, has a low proportion (15%) staying longer than 3 days. This may indicate that, at this time, many people were being admitted for a short period of observation. In contrast, over two-fifths (41%) of patients discharged from South Manchester had stayed over 3 days. This suggests that some of the variation we observed among districts may reflect differing local admission policies. However, this is not the whole cause of observed differences as the underlying figures based on a stay for 3 days or more display just as much variation.

Table 2.7 Comparison of incidence rates by (a) discharges from district and (b) residence in district, showing difference in rates (expressed as rates per 100 000 resident population)

District	(a)	(b)	(a–b)
Blackburn	389	623	−234
Burnley	154	259	−105
West Lancs	263	352	−89
Rochdale	223	308	−85
Trafford	88	162	−74
Oldham	309	339	−20
Blackpool	153	166	−13
Stockport	256	268	−12
Salford	169	179	−10
Bolton	156	155	1
Wigan	198	191	7
Bury	258	224	34
Tameside	263	226	37
Central Manchester	455	354	101
South Manchester	391	242	149
Lancaster	502	290	212
Chorley	568	236	332
Preston	886	530	356
North Manchester	722	356	366
Total	297	275	22

The overall level of 76 per 100 000 disguises a range of 21–230 per 100 000, which in an average district with a quarter of a million population, will mean a difference in a potential demand for rehabilitation of 52–575 people. More recently, guidelines for immediate treatment and admission have been introduced in some UK hospitals (Table 2.9). These may result in less variation than previously observed.

IS IT FEASIBLE TO PLAN FROM SUCH DATA?

What can we learn from these data? Regional figures of incidence of head injury in the North West are similar to national published estimates. However, variation in incidence at the local level suggests that such 'ball-park' figures will be of little value for planning services at the local level. Only one in five of the districts in the North West Region in the UK had an incidence which was within 20% of the regional incidence or national estimate! Interdistrict flows are clearly substantial in some areas and these will affect the location of acute rehabilitation services. The likelihood of admission may also be a function of varying local admissions policy, although underlying more serious injury requiring a stay of 3 or more days is just as variable.

Table 2.8 Discharges after at least 3 days stay following head injury by district and sex of patient (expressed as sex-specific and total rates per 100 000 resident population, together with percentage of all patients discharged in 1986)

| District | Sex | | | 3 days as % |
	Male	Female	All	of all patients
Trafford	26	16	21	24
Tameside	44	39	41	16
Burnley	72	29	50	32
Bolton	69	33	50	32
Salford	77	28	52	31
Wigan	60	46	53	27
Blackburn	71	44	57	15
Blackpool	86	37	60	39
Bury	90	35	62	24
Stockport	79	53	65	25
Oldham	75	59	67	22
Rochdale	87	50	68	30
West Lancs	93	67	80	30
Chorley	109	79	94	17
Central Manchester	156	64	108	24
Lancaster	148	87	116	23
South Manchester	239	82	160	41
Preston	294	168	229	26
North Manchester	333	133	230	32
Total	100	53	76	26

Despite the current emphasis in some countries on independent smaller units delivering health care, planning to meet the rehabilitation needs of those who have had a head injury ought to be done with a clear picture of the variation in demand at the regional level. Such planning has to take account of all the factors discussed above. It needs to take into account the variation in incidence by discharge district and among residents of each district and, if possible, the variation in more

Table 2.9 Criteria for hospital admission after head injury (data by kind permission of Mr John Sloan FRCS, Consultant in Accident and Emergency, Leeds General Infirmary)

- Depressed conscious level
- Prolonged amnesia or history of more than brief coma at site
- Fits, vomiting (more than twice) or severe headache
- Focal neurological signs
- Skull fracture
- Alcohol plus head injury
- Patient would be alone if returned home

severe injuries. Supplementary data to enable a focus on actual brain injury will obviously enhance the planning process, but care needs to be taken to ensure that the underlying quality of data is good enough to support this.

Knowledge of the underlying sociodemographic structure of the population will also help understand differences in demand. Work done by the UK Office of Population Censuses and Surveys allows an examination of incidence in the North West Region by the socioeconomic classification of its districts [21]. Table 2.10 shows that the variation in incidence within socioeconomic group is variable, but overall not that large.

Table 2.10 Comparison of incidence rates by socioeconomic classification (discharges by residence in district per 100 000 resident population and age–sex standardized rates)

Classification	District	Rate	Standardized
Established high-status	Trafford	162	164
	Stockport	268	271
Higher-status growth	Chorley	236	332
	West Lancs	352	345
Resort and retirement	Blackpool	166	182
	Lancaster	290	312
Mixed town and country	Wigan	191	190
	Bury	224	225
	Tameside	226	227
Traditional manufacturing	Bolton	155	152
	Burnley	259	256
	Rochdale	308	297
	Oldham	339	339
	Central Manchester	354	342
	Preston	530	527
	Blackburn	623	615
Service centres and cities	Salford	179	185
	South Manchester	242	244
	North Manchester	356	361
Total		275	–

The greatest variation occurs in the traditional manufacturing areas, which were most vulnerable to change in the recession in the UK of the early 1980s. Elsewhere rates were very similar, usually differing by less than a magnitude of two which, as there was an overall variation in rates by a factor of four, suggests some clustering by socioeconomic group. This lends support to the data presented above showing that as well as age and gender, social and economic aspects also contribute to variation.

CONCLUSION

It is possible to imagine two quite distinct districts: one rural, working locally, predominately middle-aged or retired, with one dominant ethnic grouping; the other might be an inner-city district, a large centre of employment, with a predominately young population of mixed ethnic origin. Both these districts would be ill-served by using national or regional figures for incidence, even if these were of actual brain damage, to plan their rehabilitation services.

Proper planning depends upon accurate case ascertainment, is based on accurate data and demands an understanding of the complex flow of people in and out of districts, along with the underlying socioeconomic characteristics of those districts.

REFERENCES

1. Servadei F, Bastianelli S, Naccarato G et al. Epidemiology and sequelae of head injury in San Marino. *Journal of Neurosurgical Sciences* 1985; **29**: 297–303.
2. Lyle DM, Quine S, Bauman A et al. Counting heads: estimating traumatic brain injury in New South Wales. *Community Health Studies* 1990; **14**: 118–125.
3. Servadei F, Ciucci G, Piazza G et al. A prospective clinical and epidemiological study of head injuries in northern Italy: the Commune of Ravenna. *Italian Journal of Neurological Sciences* 1988; **9**: 449–457.
4. Engberg AW, Biering-Sorensen F. Occurrence of traumatic brain injury in Denmark illustrated by hospital statistics. *Ugeskrift for Laeger* 1990; **153**: 16–21.
5. Brookes M, MacMillan R, Cully S et al. Head injuries in accident and emergency departments. How different are children from adults? *Journal of Epidemiology and Community Health* 1990; **44**: 147–151.
6. Nell V, Brown DSO. Epidemiology of traumatic brain injury in Johannesburg: II. Morbidity, mortality and etiology. *Social Science and Medicine* 1991; **33**: 289–296.
7. Tiret L, Hausherr E, Thicoipe M et al. The Epidemiology of head trauma in Aquitaine (France), 1986: a community-based study of hospital admissions and deaths. *International Journal of Epidemiology* 1990; **19**: 133–140.
8. Nestvold K, Lundar T, Blikra G. Head injuries during one year in a central hospital in Norway: a prospective study. Epidemiologic features. *Neuroepidemiology* 1988; **7**: 134–144.
9. Jagger J, Levine JI, Jane JA et al. Epidemiologic features of head injury in a predominantly rural population. *Journal of Trauma* 1984; **24**: 40–44.
10. Edna TH, Cappelen J. Hospital admitted head injury. A prospective study in Trondelag, Norway, 1979–1980. *Scandinavian Journal of Social Medicine* 1985; **13**: 23–27.
11. Annoni JM, Beer S, Kesselring J. Folgen des schweren Schaedel-Hirn-Traumas: eine epidemiologische Studie im Kanton St Gallen. *Schweizerische Medizinische Wochenschrift* 1991; **121**: 207–213. In: *Disability and Rehabilitation* 1992; **14**(1): 23–26.
12. Kraus JF, Black MA, Hessol N et al. The incidence of acute brain injury and serious impairment in a defined population. *American Journal of Epidemiology* 1984; **119**: 186–201.

13. Fife D, Faich G, Hollinshead W *et al*. Incidence and outcome of hospital-treated head injury in Rhode Island. *American Journal of Public Health* 1986; **76**: 773–778.
14. World Health Organization (WHO). *International Classification of Diseases, Injuries, and Causes of Death*, 9th revision. Geneva: World Health Organization, 1979.
15. Hill AB. *Principles of Medical Statistics*. New York: Oxford University Press, 1961.
16. Whitman S, Coonley-Hoganson R, Desai BT. Comparative head trauma experiences in two socioeconomically different area communities: Chicago – a population study. *American Journal of Epidemiology* 1984; **119**: 570–580.
17. Horowitz I, Costeff H, Sadan N *et al*. Childhood head injuries in Israel: epidemiology and outcome. *International Rehabilitation Medicine*, 1983; **5**: 32–36.
18. Viazquez-Barquero A, Sanz F, Montiaga F *et al*. Epidemiology and course of craniocerebral injuries in children in Cantabria. *Neurologia* 1990; **5**: 155–159.
19. Annergers JF, Grabow JD, Kurland LT *et al*. The incidence, causes, and secular trends of head trauma in Olmsted County, Minnesota, 1935–1974. *Neurology* 1980; **30**: 912–919.
20. Warnock H. Northin D, Carberry S *et al*. Head injury: developing community occupational therapy to meet the challenge. *British Journal of Occupational Therapy*, 1992; **55**: 99–102.
21. Craig J. *A 1981 Socio-economic Classification of Local and Health Authorities of Great Britain. Office of Population Censuses and Surveys*. London: HMSO, 1985.

A national service:
coma to community

3

Zeev Groswasser

INTRODUCTION

Until recently, the fate of patients with traumatic brain injury (TBI) was gloomy. It was assumed, that once they survived the acute state, nothing more could be done, despite their normal estimated life expectancy, especially in cases of penetrating brain lesions [1–4] uncomplicated by post-traumatic epilepsy. Conroy and Kraus [4] summarized their experience by stating that 'people [with TBI] who are discharged alive from the hospital have survival comparable to that of the population they came from'.

Rehabilitation medicine was introduced in the western world after the Second World War, when attention was focused on the fate of handicapped soldiers and later on handicapped people in general. It took almost another 25 years, until the late 1960s and early 1970s, for the discipline to include TBI patients. Today, TBI is one of the leading topics in rehabilitation medicine. In Israel, the deep interest in TBI patients was stirred somewhat earlier because of the 1956 Sinai Campaign and the 1967 Six Day War. There were few guidelines available at that time on the care of TBI veterans with blunt and penetrating lesions, so it was the rehabilitation staff at Loewenstein Rehabilitation Hospital (LRH) that took up the gauntlet. LRH is a non-profit institute of the National Sick Fund of the Labour Federation of Israel, which currently covers over 70% of the national population. It was established in the early 1940s for rehabilitation of victims of work accidents who required long-term convalescence. A number of British Second World War veterans were also treated here. During the 1960s, especially after the Six Day War, all soldiers suffering from TBI were referred to LRH. Thereafter, with the rapid increase in motorization of the country, civilian victims of road accidents also began to be referred in increasing numbers. However, it took the Yom Kippur War in 1973 for the Ministries of Health and Defence to designate LRH the national centre for treatment of all TBI patients. LRH is today affiliated with the Sackler Faculty of Medicine in Tel Aviv University and is deeply involved also in training of undergraduates and postgraduate medical and paramedical students. Besides its practical interest in TBI, LRH staff had a strong academic interest in the structure–function relationship within the central nervous system. This question became pivotal in the mid-1960s, when the books of A. R. Luria were translated into English and neuropsychology became an established field for the assessment and, later, treatment of cognitive disorders.

The introduction of computerized tomography and magnetic resonance imaging furthered interest in TBI and enabled a better understanding of the nature and extent of brain damage at the acute phase as well as at later phases of the rehabilitation process. Intensive care management immensely improved the survival rate of patients with brain trauma, resulting in more patients with severe disabilities and handicaps not encountered in the past. Initially, it was virtually impossible to compare results among different centres because the definitions even of commonly used terms such as coma, stupor and delirium were poorly defined and were interpreted differently by various authors. The Glasgow Coma Scale, introduced by Teasdale and Jennett in 1974 [5], was instrumental in the formation of a well-delineated, common language that enabled comparison of various treatment methods for patients with common grades of brain trauma. In 1975, Jennett and Bond published the Glasgow Outcome Scale for assessment of late recovery from TBI, which was another important landmark in the evolution of late evaluation of TBI patients.

DOMAINS OF TBI

TBI affects four main domains of human activity: 1) motor behaviour; 2) communication disorders; 3) cognitive deficits and 4) changes in behaviour and personality. It is only brain trauma that can cause such profound changes. It has been shown that the late outcome of TBI patients is governed by the status of these domains [6–9]. Besides brain injury, 58% of affected patients also have trauma to other parts of the body. Whenever two or more sites, apart from the brain, are involved, a more severe brain insult is indicated, and outcome is relatively poorer [10].

GOALS OF TBI REHABILITATION

Victims of this so-called 'silent epidemic' [11] of modern life are usually young adults. Almost 75% of TBI patients in Israel are 15–29 years old, three-quarters of these male. These are the years during which the educational, professional and occupational foundations of life are normally laid; the time when people start families, forge careers and become responsible members of the community. Severe TBI disrupts this life, severs the social links of the victims and makes them unfit to continue in their previous occupation. It is the aim of the rehabilitation process to restore as far as possible the social and occupational integration of these patients. The measurement and quantification of social—occupational reintegration are the subject of considerable debate. Jennett and Bond [12] considered return to work unrealistic for severe TBI patients and Rao et al. [13] raised serious doubts regarding the usefulness of the Glasgow Outcome Scale in a rehabilitation setting. It is obvious, however, that solutions to this question are closely tied to the cultural and socioeconomic background of the patients, and there may therefore be many different answers. Melamed et al. [14] showed that, in Israeli society, the ability of adult TBI patients to maintain a work position (or for children to return to school) is highly correlated with patient's subjective evaluation of the quality of life, as measured by the Rehabilitation Need and Status Scale [15]. We believe that, given the fear of unemployment and the established links between unemployment and health, the state of post-injury employment could serve as a reliable integrative aim for rehabilitation outcome in Israel and other Western countries.

This view of the key role of employment status in TBI patient outcome is supported in several recent publications. A British committee set up to study the aftercare of head-injured patients [16] concluded that 'returning to work is regarded as a major aim for brain-damaged patients'. Lezak [17] stressed the role of work in restructuring life and in providing stability and purpose. Stanbrook et al. [18] concluded that vocational rehabilitation is an essential and realistic component in a holistic rehabilitation program.

ADMISSION POLICY

Our definition of the four major domains of brain damage provides a general picture as to what should be treated, but questions of who should be admitted to the rehabilitation programme and at what stage remain open. The approach varies among different centres. Some institutes admit only patients who are fully conscious and independent in daily living activities. The policy at LRH is to allow even severe TBI patients a chance, because no method has yet been devised to determine with certainty the fate of patients who are still in coma or who have just recovered consciousness, a few days or weeks after trauma. Patients in the latter stage may be confused, agitated and disorientated but in otherwise stable physical condition. Thus, they become a burden on intensive care units or neurosurgical wards, which may lead to a decrease in the quality of nursing and medical care they receive and they may develop bedsores and contractures. LRH has a special intensive care unit of 16 beds to which unconscious TBI patients from all over the country are admitted. Once they regain consciousness and establish purposeful and meaningful contact with the staff they are transferred directly to the Brain Injury Rehabilitation Department. It should be stressed that, if the patient is able to communicate with family members, but not with staff members, he is admitted to the coma unit. He must have contact with the staff before his transfer to the rehabilitation department so that he can conduct a meaningful dialogue with them, which is the base for further therapy.

The in-patient brain injury service has a capacity of 48 beds for adults and 15 beds for children. The children's unit has additional services, such as special education, financed by the local authority and the Ministry of Education and Culture. Patients are admitted to the department without prior examination by anyone on the LRH team. For the sake of proper continuity of care, they are asked to bring with them copies of their brain CT scans and any other relevant medical data. The duration of unconsciousness has an important relation to late vocational outcome and may be used to assess severity of TBI. Groswasser and Sazbon [19] showed that only about 11% of patients who were unconscious longer than one month were able to maintain a self-supporting work position at the end of the rehabilitation process. In a recent study, coma duration showed a significant correlation with vocational placement (Spearman $r = 0.45$) while, interestingly, age did not [20]. Other authors have used the duration of post-traumatic amnesia (PTA) as a yardstick for measuring the severity of TBI. We believe, however, that the latter cannot always be ascertained with precision and, therefore, we ascertain during the admission process the exact duration of unconsciousness.

ADMISSION PROCEDURE

Patients come with a close family member because often patients themselves are unable to provide the necessary information. Patients undergo a complete physical and neurological examination while family members are interviewed by nurses, social workers, speech therapists and psychologists, so that the treating staff may have the widest view possible of the patients' habits, familial, social and occupational background and formal and informal academic achievements. The procedure serves to familiarize concerned family members with the team and to obtain, sometimes for the first time since the trauma, a more general idea about what to expect from the patient, how to behave towards him and how to react to his behaviour. Their prior information in these areas is often inadequate, and insight into what the patient is going through is lacking.

The assessment of the patient enables the staff to form, within a short time, a detailed picture of his physical and neurobehavioural deficits and to set short- and long-term goals. It must be stressed that the team approach is patient-orientated; that is, one patient who may have many problems in different fields is treated by various team members as a whole person. There may be a certain amount of overlap of information and sometimes even treatment, but this is preferable to the risk of 'blank' areas in the rehabilitation programme.

INTEGRATIVE APPROACH TO PSYCHODYNAMIC ASPECTS OF TBI

During the recovery process, TBI patients manifest a wide spectrum of behavioural changes. We studied the nature of these psychodynamic changes to improve our understanding of what takes place in the TBI patient and thereby form an integrative approach within a supportive milieu [21]. TBI patients, once awake, are often disorientated in time and space. They do not know where they are or what has happened to them. They must recover their past and learn to live in an entirely different situation from the one they were used to before sustaining trauma. They ask themselves questions like, 'Who am I?' and 'What is going on?'. Even if answers are provided, they cannot establish any sort of continuity in their life, because their retrograde and/or anterograde memory may be severely impaired. They also, usually, have a decreased ability to process information and, because of the disturbances in thought processes, are unable to make any sense of their present situation. These difficulties may be expressed physically by psychomotor restlessness. Patients may have problems expressing themselves, because of communication disorders (speech and/or language), and may appear confused. The world may be conceived as demanding, even hostile, and as a result the patients feel they cannot rely on or trust even close, familiar figures who are good, protecting and warm. Although they have to relearn their entire past within a short time, childish behaviour is not tolerated, because they are outwardly adults. Besides the mental problems, they might also suffer from physical disabilities, causing them to feel that they cannot control even their body any more. Thus, early phase TBI patients are uncooperative, totally dependent on a misunderstood external world. They are in an extremely anxious or even catastrophic state (in the psychiatric sense) and may respond, in defence, with extreme aggression. This phase may last up to a few weeks. Some patients will later describe this early recovery phase as a dream state. Some can pinpoint the moment at which they realized that they were in a real situation; for others, it fades out gradually. The termination of this phase sometimes coincides with the end of the post-traumatic amnesia and can mark a turning point in the rehabilitation process. Why some patients exhibit this sharp point in the recovery process while others do not is not well understood. Therapy at this stage aims at rebuilding patients' basic trust with the outside world.

The environment should be sympathetic but not permissive. That includes the family. If such patients are sent home directly from the general hospital without the family receiving advice with regard to restructuring their environment, it may be difficult at a later stage to break bad habits formed now and reshape abnormal behaviour. It is therefore recommended that such patients be referred to specialized rehabilitation centres at the earliest opportunity. Recent data by Mackay *et al.* [22] have shown the beneficial effects of early rehabilitative intervention in TBI patients. Our clinical impression is that patients who exhibit psychomotor restlessness at the early phase after recovering consciousness will have an improved outcome over those who show marked passivity and apathy [23]. Some patients, although still in a confused state, demand to go home. If there is no other interfering medical problem, patients may be sent home for a day or even a weekend. Here, family cooperation is especially important, because the family has to be instructed to allow them only one visitor at a time, with breaks between visitors. This will ensure the ability of patients to cope adequately within a known background. Once the patients have renewed contact with their previously known environment and have seen that they are not rejected by family and friends, they are likely to become better orientated and more cooperative.

THERAPY

The complexity of TBI indicates a need for a multidisciplinary rehabilitation team with a patient-orientated approach. As time passes, the key problems of the patient change; during the more acute earlier phase medical and physical problems dominate, whereas at later phases neuropsychological, behavioural, vocational and social problems come to the fore. This span of problems, treated by different types of professional over the years, creates theoretical and practical management needs. The team must be well coordinated and balanced to be able to decide what best to do and when, and to establish continuity of follow-up and treatment. It is our experience that physicians knowledgeable in the neurological and neurobehavioural aspects of central nervous system (CNS) function are the best long-term choice for coordinating and balancing patients' changing needs. Other team members may serve as individual case managers. It is beyond the scope of the present chapter to describe specific therapeutic techniques, but a few comments about the training of some team members are presented.

Over half the patients referred to rehabilitation services in Israel suffer mainly from functional disabilities because of CNS lesions of either vascular or traumatic origin. As a result, physicians are heavily exposed to problems that stem from CNS damage and recovery. Special attention has been placed in recent years on postgraduate training of physicians in physical medicine and rehabilitation (PMR), including basic and advanced courses in neuropsychology, speech and language disorders, functional brain models and plasticity. Training in occupational therapy has changed remarkably as well and today includes similar courses. These reforms have created a wide base of therapists with improved understanding of CNS function and its relation with the problems of TBI patients, so that, although independence in activities of daily living is still an important early goal in occupational therapy, more emphasis is now placed on cognitive assessment and training. New tools, such as the Loewenstein Occupational Therapy Cognitive Assessment (LOTCA), have been developed and standardized [24,25], enabling early, rapid and accurate assessment of cognitive problems. Therapy aimed at specific problems can therefore be started at an earlier phase, even before detailed and comprehensive neuropsychological evaluations are conducted. Other integral aspects of the work performed by occupational therapists at LRH are prevocational training and early vocational assessment. Both occupational therapists and neuropsychologists use specific computer-based cognitive training schemes. The long-term beneficial effects of these programmes were shown by Evyatar et al. [26].

DISCHARGE PROCEDURE AND OUTCOME

The decision to discharge a TBI patient rests on successful integration of the patient's achievements, his mental state, the attitude of his family and the existence of an adequate post-hospitalization programme. The recovery phase of severe TBI patients stretches over months and even years. Therefore the treating staff tend to prolong patients' hospitalization so that the patients may benefit as much as possible. However, some patients, after being in hospital for a few months, are afraid of facing unsupported situations; they develop symptoms of over-hospitalization and are afraid to leave the sheltered environment of the hospital. Conversely, others lack insight into their problems, refuse therapy and ask to leave the hospital as soon as possible. Discharge, however, signifies a crucial point in the process of recovery and must be carefully planned. Social reintegration, which is the final goal of the rehabilitation process, starts with the family; it is almost impossible to rehabilitate severe TBI patients who have no family. As already mentioned, we have found that structured weekend home visits help both patients and their family adapt to the new state. If patients have been previously engaged in gainful employment, a thorough check is done to determine whether they can resume their pre-trauma position. This includes complete assessment of residual physical and neurobehavioural deficits as well as job demands. If their return to work is a real possibility, their permission is obtained to call in the employer. It is not unusual for patients to begin employment at the worksite on a part-time basis while still officially hospitalized, using the remainder of their time to clarify and settle related problems that arise. This interim period is also used for dealing with employers' fears, to assure them that the patient in question is fully capable of performing the job. On many occasions after discharge, patients hold a job part-time for a couple of weeks and thereafter gradually progress to full-time. They are closely followed during this period and are able to get in touch with the staff whenever they need advice. In consideration of the integral part played by vocational training and placement in TBI rehabilitation, and the fact that most TBI patients are young adult males, many of whom have just finished their studies and have no previous working experience, a vocational training centre was built on the campus of LRH in 1982. Here, patients can be trained on an individual basis at their own pace.

Those who pass the government-issued examination at termination of the program receive official certification in their field. In addition, patients are taught methods of finding and applying for employment. Graduates are closely followed for long periods, and any problem that arises on the part of the trainee or the employer is dealt with almost immediately. Vocational rehabilitation may be started for some patients even while they are still hospitalized. On that occasion staff members from the Vocational Rehabilitation Centre are called in to join the team, enabling direct contact and flow of information among the team members. If a patient is scheduled to continue pre-injury studies, careful attention is given to create conditions that will ensure a gradual increase in the workload. Individual assistance is provided as necessary, at least at the beginning. These patients are followed at short intervals at the out-patient clinic and encouraged to consult team members, officially and unofficially, whenever they need to. Some continue cognitive and supportive therapy on a regular basis for long periods.

Close family members of TBI patients are also encouraged to consult team members after discharge. Studies have shown that over half (50–66%) the severe TBI patients who attended comprehensive rehabilitation programmes were able to resume their previous work positions or equivalent ones [6,9,13]. Johnson [27] stressed the time element in returning to work; his conclusions were that the chances to do so are good within the first 2 years after trauma and thereafter decrease dramatically. About 30%

of severe TBI patients are unable to undertake regular jobs, but are, nevertheless, independent in activities of daily living and reside with their families. Some are referred to intensive day centres for extended periods of training and education, to improve cognitive functions and social skills and for eventual referral to sheltered workshops. Melamed *et al* [14] found that patients who maintain positions under sheltered conditions consider themselves as having a fair quality of life and are better adjusted socially [28] than those who do not work at all.

About 15–20% of severe TBI patients are unemployable, even under sheltered conditions. Most of these patients were unconscious for prolonged periods and were left with severe physical and neurobehavioural deficits. Some are taken home by relatives, and others are sent to nursing homes. A small percentage continue to improve over the years, especially from the physical aspect, but their residual communicative, cognitive and behavioural deficits render any sort of employment unrealistic, even in the long term.

FOLLOW-UP TREATMENT AND ASSESSMENT OF OUTCOME

Brain-injured patients and their families need long-term care and support. With regard to family support, studies have shown that, at 3 months after patients suffer trauma, female relatives manifest significant psychiatric morbidity at a level concomitant with the severity of the injury and function poorly in social roles associated with the home [29]. Brooks *et al.* [30] found that the psychiatric symptoms of relatives of severe TBI patients were worse 1 year after injury and that family members were under great strain and constant anxiety. Day centres and other extended forms of care have been shown to contribute to the quality of survival as assessed by the patients themselves. One-third of patients reported cognitive improvement and almost half felt that they had achieved better behavioural control, which positively affected their family life and, to a lesser degree, their social life [9,31]. However, it has been found that, at 6 months after discharge TBI, patients are doing less well than expected by the in-patient facility at discharge. This is most probably due to a combination of unrealistic team expectations and poor patient acceptance of disability [32]. Thus, the existence of a follow-up mechanism for later intervention, to assist the patient in changing directions, is a mandatory element of the rehabilitation programme.

RECOMMENDATIONS AND SUMMARY

The rehabilitation of TBI patients is a complex process for which a well-integrated, multidisciplinary, patient-orientated team is needed. Flow of information among staff members, as well as between staff and family, must be constant in order to establish an environment of trust among all participants and improve patient rehabilitation. The patient and his family are regarded as partners in the process. Social–occupational reintegration is the ultimate goal of therapy, and actual employment can serve as an integrative objective criterion of successful rehabilitation. Unemployed patients who nevertheless live an active life, also subjectively report a good quality of life [32]. The LRH experience, which is essentially a national experience, indicates the great benefit of large rehabilitation centres. They enable a well-trained, multidisciplinary team to be built up to provide the continuous non-fragmented care so necessary for these patients and their families.

REFERENCES

1. Weiss GH, Caveness WF, Einsiedel-Lechtape H *et al*. Life expectancy and causes of death in a group of head-injured veterans of World War I. *Archives of Neurology* 1982; **39**: 741–743.
2. Rish BL, Daniel Dillon J, Weiss GH. Mortality following penetrating craniocerebral injury. An analysis of death of the Vietnam Head Injury Registry population. *Journal of Neurosurgery* 1983; **59**: 775–780.
3. Corkin S, Sullivan EV, Carr FA. Prognostic factors for life expectancy after penetrating head injury. *Archives of Neurology* 1984; **41**: 975–977.
4. Conroy C, Kraus JF. Survival after brain injury. Cause of death, length of survival, and prognostic variables in a cohort of brain-injured people. *Neuroepidemiology* 1988; **7**: 13–22.
5. Teasdale G, Jennett B. Assessment of coma and impaired consciousness: a practical scale. *Lancet* 1974; **2**: 81–84.
6. Najenson T, Mendelson L, Schechter I *et al*. (1974) Rehabilitation after severe head injury. *Scandinavian Journal of Rehabilitation Medicine* 1974; **6**: 5–12.
7. Najenson T, Groswasser Z, Stern JM *et al*. Prognostic factors in rehabilitation after severe head injury. *Scandinavian Journal of Rehabilitation Medicine* 1975; 7: 101_105.
8. Groswasser Z, Mendelson L, Stern JM *et al*. Re-evaluation of prognostic parameters in rehabilitation after severe head injury. *Scandinavian Journal of Rehabilitation Medicine*, 1977; **9**: 147–149.
9. Najenson T, Groswasser Z, Mendelson L *et al*. Rehabilitation outcome of brain damaged patients after severe head injury. *International Rehabilitation Medicine* 1980; **2**: 17–22.
10. Groswasser Z, Cohen M, Blankstein E. Polytrauma associated with traumatic brain injury: incidence, nature and impact on rehabilitation outcome. *Brain Injury* 1990; **4**: 161–166.
11. Goldstein M. Traumatic brain injury: a silent epidemic. *Annals of Neurology* 1990; **27**: 327.
12. Jennett B, Bond M. Assessment of outcome after severe brain damage. A practical scale. *Lancet* 1975; **1**: 480–484.
13. Rao N, Rosenthal M, Cronin-Stubb D *et al*. Return to work after rehabilitation following traumatic brain injury. *Brain Injury* 1990; **4**: 49–56.

14. Melamed S, Stern JM, Rahmani L *et al.* Work congruence, behaviourial pathology and rehabilitation status of severe craniocerebral injury. In: Lahav M, ed. *Psychological Research in Rehabilitation.* Tel-Aviv: Ministry of Defence Publishing House, 1982: pp 59–74.
15. Kravetz S. Rehabilitation need and status: substance, structure and process. Unpublished PhD thesis, University of Wisconsin, 1973.
16. The Aftercare of Brain Injury with emphasis on inter-professional co-operation and guidelines for the future. Meeting held at The Royal College of Physicians. 13 November 1987.
17. Lezak MD. Psychological implications of traumatic brain damage of the patient's family. *Rehabilitation Psychology* 1986; **31**: 241–250.
18. Stanbrook M, Moore AD, Deviane *et al.* Effects of mild, moderate and severe head injury on long-term vocational status. *Brain Injury* 1990; **4**: 183–190.
19. Groswasser Z, Sazbon L. Outcome of 134 patients with prolonged post-traumatic unawareness. II. Functional outcome of 72 patients recovering consciousness. *Journal of Neurosurgery* 1990; **72**: 81–84.
20. Reider-Groswasser I, Cohen M, Costeff H *et al.* Late CT findings in brain trauma: relationship to cognitive and behavioural sequelae and to vocational outcome. *American Journal of Roentgenology* 1993; **160**: 147–152.
21. Groswasser Z, Stern JM. *Dynamic Cognitive and Behavioural Changes During the Rehabilitation Process of Traumatic Brain Injury.* IRMA Monograph Series. Israel: International Rehabilitation Medical Association, 1989.
22. Mackay LE, Bernstein BA, Chapman PE *et al.* Early intervention in severe head injury: long-term benefits of formalized program. *Archives of Physical Medicine and Rehabilitation* 1992; **73**: 635–641.
23. Stern JM, Melamed S, Silberg S *et al.* Behaviourial disturbances as an expression of severity of cerebral damage. *Scandinavian Journal of Rehabilitation Medicine* 1985; **Supp 12**: 36–41.
24. Najenson T, Rahmani R, Elazar B *et al.* An elementary cognitive assessment and treatment of the craniocerebral injured patient. In: Edelstein BA, Couture EG, eds. *Behavioural Assessment and Rehabilitation of the Traumatically Brain-Damaged.* New York: Plenum Press, 1984: pp 313–338.
25. Katz N, Itzkovich M, Averbuch S *et al.* Loewenstein Occupational Therapy Cognitive Assessment (LOTCA) Battery for brain injured patients: reliability and validity. *American Journal of Occupational Therapy* 1989; **43**: 184–192.
26. Evyatar A, Stern MJ, Shem-Tov M *et al.* Hypothesis forming and computerized cognitive therapy. In: Wood R, Fussy I, eds. *Cognitive Rehabilitation in Perspective.* London: Taylor & Francis, 1990: pp 147–163.
27. Johnson R. Return to work after severe head injury. *International Rehabilitation Studies* 1987; **9**: 44–49.
28. Katz S, Galatzer A, Kravetz S. The physical, psycho-social and vocational effectiveness of a sheltered workshop for brain-damaged war veterans. In: Lahav M, ed. *Psychological Research in Rehabilitation.* Tel-Aviv: Ministry of Defence Publishing House, 1982: pp 75–85.
29. Livingstone MG, Brooks ND, Bond M. Three months after head injury: psychiatric and social impact on relatives. *Journal of Neurology, Neurosurgery and Psychiatry* 1985; **48**: 870–875.
30. Brooks ND, Campsie L, Symington C *et al.* The five year outcome of severe blunt head injury: a relative's view. *Journal of Neurology, Neurosurgery, and Psychiatry* 1986; **49**: 764–770.

31. Stern JM, Groswasser Z, Alis R *et al*. Day centre experience in rehabilitation of craniocerebral injured patients. *Scandinavian Journal of Rehabilitation Medicine* 1985; **Supp 12**: 53–59.
32. Melamed S, Groswasser Z, Stern MJ. Acceptance of disability, work involvement and subjective rehabilitation status of traumatic brain injured (TBI) patients. *Brain Injury* 1992; **6**: 233–243.

A regional service:
developing a head injury service

4

Mike Barnes

WHY A REGIONAL SERVICE?

Ideally, rehabilitation after an acute head injury should be carried out as near to the injured person's home as possible, and the later stages of rehabilitation should be within the home and with the active involvement of family and carers. So why do we need a regional head injury rehabilitation service at all? The numbers of head-injured people with moderate and severe injuries are probably sufficient to generate a viable district rehabilitation unit (about 65 people per annum in a typical English health district with a population of 250 000 [1]). However, it is highly unlikely that any health district will be able to find sufficient therapy and neuropsychology expertise to cope with the complex and wide ranging impairments and disabilities that can occur after head injury. This is particularly true in the postacute stage of recovery, when a complicated range of physical disabilities is often compounded by major cognitive and behavioural disturbance. At times of community re-entry and for ongoing support then local schemes are preferable. However, for the first few months after severe and moderate injuries, specialist regional units are necessary both for the rehabilitation process itself and also to act as centres for education, training and research.

IDEAL REQUIREMENTS FOR A REGIONAL HEAD INJURY SERVICE

PROXIMITY TO REGIONAL NEUROSURGICAL SERVICE

Any head injury rehabilitation unit should have close liaison and a good working relationship with neurosurgical colleagues. Ideally, a rehabilitation team should have access to the head-injured person and his/her family as soon as possible after the injury. There are a number of reasons why this is necessary. Firstly, the rehabilitation team will have the expertise to advise on positioning and stretching, in order to minimize unnecessary complications of spasticity, particularly contractures. A speech therapist and dietician may need to advise on the management of swallowing disorders, nasogastric or gastrostomy feeding. A neuropsychologist may be invaluable to advise staff on the appropriate management of behavioural problems that are so common during the period of post-traumatic amnesia. Secondly, members of the team may be best placed to offer guidance, reassurance and information regarding head injury and appropriate honest advice with regard to prognosis, albeit that any accurate guide to prognosis is virtually impossible in the very early stages. Finally, the patient and family can get to know the rehabilitation staff and visit the unit, so that the eventual transfer from the neurosurgical service to the rehabilitation unit can be as smooth as possible. The team, in consultation with the neurosurgeons, will be able to advise on the best time for transfer, which, in my opinion, should be as early as possible after head injury once medical and surgical stability has been achieved [2].

PHYSICAL BASE

Does a regional head injury service require a physical base? It would be possible for a team based within a hospital to support patients directly on medical or surgical wards. However, there are advantages in the creation of a specific rehabilitation unit. Wade *et al.* [3] summarize the advantages of stroke rehabilitation units within a district general hospital setting. The same benefits apply to a head injury unit: the physical structure could be made more conducive to rehabilitation; the team approach is facilitated; staff morale should be higher; research should be stimulated; voluntary help is more likely; record keeping and follow-up (and thus audit) are more easily managed. Unfortunately, there are no studies that compare the roving team approach to that of a team based within a rehabilitation unit, but most reports recommend the latter [4–7]. The geographical site of the rehabilitation unit is probably less important than the internal design. However, there are advantages in moving from an acute hospital setting to a separate rehabilitation unit, which is more readily seen as a step towards return to the community. Appropriate design can be facilitated on a separate site; it is difficult to fulfil the requirements of both an acute ward and a rehabilitation unit with the same design. It is axiomatic that rehabilitation units should be fully accessible both internally and by public transport. Ideally a unit should be within a local community, in order to allow the individual to be introduced to a real community environment. The internal design should facilitate independence and should preferably include single rooms, accessible kitchens, dining facilities, large and small day rooms and space to allow spouse and family to stay with or near the patient and thus participate in the rehabilitation process.

SIZE

What size? The number of beds needed in a regional rehabilitation unit is a very difficult question. This will depend on the population served, admission and discharge policy of the unit and age criteria. Obviously, it will also depend on whether the unit is specifically geared to head injury or whether it acts as a regional unit for people with other diagnoses and disabilities. If the unit does not have age limitations and deals only with people with severe head injuries, then a typical regional unit, serving a population of approximately 3 million people (as is the case with regional health authorities in England), would need to cater for approximately 240 people per annum [1]. If one assumes an average length of stay of approximately 8 weeks, then the unit will need to have approximately 40 beds. In the UK there are no units with that number of beds exclusively serving people with head injury.

There is a strong case for providing a separate paediatric unit. Children with head injury are very badly served in the UK. The expertise required is slightly different and obviously will need additional input from paediatric and educational specialists. It is obviously inappropriate for children to be housed in the same unit as adults, particularly as those adults are often disturbed and aggressive. There is a further case for differentiating between the 'typical' young head-injured, often male, individual and the rather more vulnerable elderly head-injured person. If separate units are not possible, then different areas in the same unit are desirable.

ASSOCIATION WITH OTHER SPECIALIST SERVICES

It is highly unlikely that the specialist services required by a head injury unit would be available specifically for that unit. A head injury unit will need to draw upon facilities and expertise of other specialist rehabilitation services that are required at a Regional level. There have been a number of reports on this subject [4,8,9] and it is generally agreed that, among other services, the following services are required:

- specialist service for complex wheelchair and special seating requirements;
- bioengineering service;
- communication aids centre;

- information, advice and assessment service with regard to car driving;
- prosthetic service;
- service for people with brain damage who have a combination of physical, psychological and severe behavioural problems;
- specialist long-term or residential facility for people in persistent vegetative state or prolonged coma.

In the real world it is easier to develop a regional neurological rehabilitation unit, which can cater for people with the most complex disabilities arising from brain and spinal cord injury, rather than a service specifically for head-injured people. Other problems are likely to include multiple sclerosis, motor neurone disease, stroke and other rarer neurological problems such as Guillain–Barré syndrome, encephalitis and severe muscular dystrophies. Such a unit could then be closely associated with the specialist services outlined above, and the whole complex could preferably be housed in a regional rehabilitation centre. However, it must be stressed that the behavioural disturbance encountered in head injury can be very disruptive and, indeed, frightening for people with other disabilities, and, whatever the configuration of the unit, a separate area should be reserved for people with behavioural problems.

ADMISSION CRITERIA

The size and scope of the unit will depend upon admission criteria. There are three major criteria to be considered: age, level of disability and whether the unit will accept postacute referrals for relatively short-term admission only or whether the unit offers a tertiary rehabilitation programme for the longer-term support of head-injured people and their families. Each criterion will have a major effect on the configuration of the unit. These decisions must be a matter of local judgement.

STAFF

This is also a vexed question. There are staffing recommendations for the UK [1,10]. Obviously the precise composition of any rehabilitation team depends on the size of the unit, admission criteria, discharge policy, availability of community support services and so on. However, it is clear that there needs to be representation from a core of disciplines – physiotherapy, occupational therapy, speech and language therapy, clinical neuropsychology, nursing, rehabilitation medicine and social work. There is a need for occasional input from a variety of other professionals such as dieticians, chiropodists, activity organizers, vocational trainers, counsellors and a variety of medical specialists on an *ad hoc* basis, particularly neurosurgeons, urologists and orthopaedic surgeons. It has been recommended in the UK [9] that the staff:patient ratios for the core disciplines are 1 : 5 for physiotherapy and occupational therapy and 1 : 20 for speech therapy, clinical psychology and social work. A 1 : 1 nurse:patient ratio is also generally accepted. There will need to be senior and junior medical staff support. The difficulty with such recommendations is that staff levels will depend on the scope and type of unit, as well as experience of the staff and the qualified/unqualified staff mix in each department. The significant danger of making such recommendations is that these serve to emphasize the departmental ethos, whereas the philosophy of rehabilitation units should be more client- than department-orientated. This problem has been overcome in some private units in the UK and more widely in the USA by the employment of rehabilitation officers/therapists, who are not attached to particular departments but are responsible to a certain number of clients/patients. The advantage of such an approach is to emphasize the patient-centred goal-setting process. The rehabilitation officer will normally be responsible for carrying out the rehabilitation process with the guidance of a smaller number of specialist therapists from relevant disciplines. The efficacy of this approach over the departmental model remains unproven. However, Eames and Wood [11] described the success of such 'role blurring' within the special circumstances of a behavioural modification unit. It is also possible that the success, at least in lay terms, of the conductive education programme in Hungary may, in part, have been due to the close therapeutic relationship of the rehabilitation therapist (conductor) with the patient.

Key worker

At the present time, in the UK it is not possible to develop the model of the rehabilitation therapist, as these individuals would need specific training and no such generic training programme exists. However, some units have developed a key worker system which goes some way towards the idea of a generic therapist. It is difficult to define a key worker, but in the context of this chapter the role of a key worker is to act as a channel of communication between the patient, family and rehabilitation team as a whole. The key worker will be the individual who is most aware of the interests, abilities and family dynamics of the patient, both before injury and during rehabilitation. The key worker, with the patient and family on the one hand and advice from therapy staff on the other, will help to determine the functional goals. He/she would act as liaison between the hospital/rehabilitation unit and the community support services to help ensure smooth transition at time of discharge. The key worker would ensure that the patient and family have ready access to information, explanation and counselling as required and provide continuity of support. The background of the key worker could be from any of the therapy disciplines, nursing or social work. There should be no reason why a cognitively intact and willing patient or family member should not act as the key worker. However, conflict can arise between the patient and the family aspirations. The key worker, if sufficiently senior in experience, can act as a useful arbitrator when such disputes arise.

OUR EXPERIENCE: HUNTERS MOOR REGIONAL REHABILITATION CENTRE

The previous paragraphs have given some general guidance on the establishment of a regional head injury unit. It may be useful to share the experience of establishing such a regional unit in Newcastle upon Tyne. The purpose of the following sections is not to illustrate the establishment of the 'ideal' unit but to give an honest appraisal of both what works well and what is not yet right in our centre.

GEOGRAPHY

The regional unit is situated in the city of Newcastle. It serves a regional population of some 3 million. There are two neurosurgical units feeding the rehabilitation unit; the larger one is in the same city, the second is approximately 50 miles to the south. Although Newcastle is a large city, the rest of the region is mainly rural, covering a large area from the Scottish border to 100 miles south and stretching 100 miles from east coast to west coast. Some districts are beginning to develop expertise in head injury rehabilitation.

THE HOSPITAL

Hunters Moor is over 100 years old, built to provide accessible residential accommodation for over 100 people with severe physical disabilities on four wards. In the early days there was much nursing and little therapy, but from the 1970s, with the coming of a more dynamic approach, more therapists and therapy space have been provided and two assessment bungalows have been built in the grounds.

DEVELOPMENT OF REGIONAL REHABILITATION SERVICE

In 1990, with help of additional funds from the regional health authority, an 18-bed rehabilitation unit was developed specifically to meet the needs of those with traumatic brain injury. Currently, 18 beds are available for rehabilitation, with another two wards providing residential and respite accommodation. A fourth ward was converted to therapy space, offices and an enlarged day unit.

ADMISSION CRITERIA

The unit has age limits of 16–65 years. The upper age limit does not cause particular problems as there is a rehabilitation service run by geriatricians in Newcastle. However, there is no specific children's brain injury service in Newcastle, and this need, although recognized, has not been met. The rehabilitation unit is not specifically for people with head injuries, but admits anyone with a severe neurological disability who could benefit from the service. About 40% of admissions are of people with moderate to severe head injury, who in turn are largely young men in the 16–30 age range. About two-thirds of admissions are male, and the main wards are mixed. There is a small, separate three-bed area for females. The bed areas are partitioned and relatively private, although such mixture of the sexes can cause problems at times, particularly when there are aggressive or disinhibited young males in residence. Recently one area has been segregated to provide a room for such individuals.

STAFFING AND KEY WORKER SYSTEM

The unit does not run a generic rehabilitation therapist model, although there is active development of a key worker system. The key worker is any professional member of staff from any background. The key worker is allocated as early as possible and, if possible, will visit the patient and family at the source of referral. The key worker is responsible for completing the various assessment and functional goal setting forms (see below) and fulfils the role outlined above. The system has generally worked well and is appreciated by staff. However, the need for regular meetings of key workers, and for initiation and ongoing training, has become apparent.

The staff within each department are as follows. These figures include unqualified staff, although in any department at least 75% of staff are qualified.

Physiotherapy	9
Occupational therapy	7
Speech therapist	2.5
Clinical neuropsychologist	2
Nursing	22
Social worker	1
Counsellor	0.5
Senior physician	1.5
Junior physician	2

These staff support the 18-bed in-patient unit, as well as servicing the day unit, which houses up to 10 individuals per day. Other staff (e.g. dietitian, chiropodist) have occasional sessional input and can be called upon on an individual referral basis. These ratios are generally sufficient to run the unit, although the balance of patients is kept under constant supervision so that a reasonable mix of disabilities and degree of behavioural disturbance is maintained. Originally there was a gross underestimate of the number of patients who would require speech therapy. It was felt that around one-third of in-patients would do so, but the figure is nearer 80%, particularly when the speech therapists are involved in swallowing assessment. The input of clinical neuropsychology is vital, and there was an original underestimate of the number of hours required from this service. The unit would benefit from an activity organizer, and extra help is needed for the social worker. It is worth noting that the unit is self-contained with regard to catering, domestic and portering staff.

We have no liaison with the Employment Rehabilitation Service, which is a major drawback.

THE SYSTEM

Admissions are prebooked and at the time of writing there is a waiting list of between 1 and 4 weeks. However, transfers are not in chronological order of referral but are determined at a weekly staff meeting according to clinical need. Once an admission is booked, a key worker is identified, who visits the patient and family. On arrival it is the key worker's responsibility to acquaint the family with the unit. The family are given an information booklet, which contains information not only about the hospital but also about their own particular problems (e.g. self-help literature produced by the National Head Injuries Association or similar literature for other diagnoses). A new admission is discussed at the weekly staff meeting and long-term and medium-term goals are determined, with particular input from the key worker. Also at this stage the first short-term (fortnightly) goals are set. The goal-setting process should be two-way between the rehabilitation team and the patient and family, although sometimes an agreement on goals is almost impossible to achieve. A case conference is called as soon as possible, so that all the team can meet together with the patient and family to discuss initial thoughts and aspirations. A second case conference is held about halfway through the projected period of stay, and a final discharge case conference is held as near to the discharge as possible. If it is possible to identify therapists and other professionals in the community, who will be dealing with the individual on discharge, then these are also contacted early and invited to the case conferences. It is sometimes difficult to get community therapists and others interested in a future client until very close to or after discharge, usually because of major workload commitments and difficulties with travelling to the regional centre. The fortnightly goals and other medium- and long-term goals are recorded on the patient's individual form, which is held by the patient or, if more convenient, by his/her key worker. There has been a tendency to change the design of the forms at regular intervals, and this has been confusing to staff and patients. A further major problem has been agreement on rating scales that should be used to monitor progress and identify problems and act as an audit and research tool. A number of accepted scales have been used in the last few years, but none seem to meet our own particular requirements for a functionally orientated scale that includes physical, psychological, behavioural and social evaluation and scoring systems. With some reluctance, because we did not wish to add to the plethora of forms already available, we have now designed our own Newcastle Independence Assessment Scale. This scale is currently being validated as part of an ongoing research project. It may have to be accepted that every unit is different and that no scale can be adequately used by a unit which has not been designed for its own purposes to suit its own requirements.

DISCHARGE AND FOLLOW-UP

The average length of stay for people with head injuries is 8 weeks. The majority of such referrals come to us approximately 4 weeks post-injury and they are thus about 3 months post-injury on discharge. The main difficulty with a regional unit is adequate liaison with the local community. In such a large geographical area this has proved a major problem, usually due to lack of appropriate staff to whom referrals can be made or because of such extreme work pressure on those staff that they cannot take referrals immediately. In an attempt to overcome this problem we have allocated our social worker and an occupational therapist to be our regional liaison team, but this has significantly reduced their time on the unit. A separate team specifically for the purpose of liaising with local therapists and following up people in the community would be ideal. After discharge from the in-patient unit, people who live reasonably locally and who can travel (either themselves, with their family or in our ambulance) can attend the day unit to continue the rehabilitation programme. Better hospital transportation to the unit is necessary, so that more people can come to this service. If patients are accepted on to the day unit programme, then the average length of stay is a further 10 weeks. The same team and the same key worker is involved with their ongoing rehabilitation at this time.

The point of final discharge may be a time of dispute. Patients must be moved on from the unit, which would otherwise take fewer admissions per annum. Often patients and family wish to continue with therapy and feel let down when discharge is discussed. The time of discharge can be very variable and, if individuals are still responding well to therapy and meeting new fortnightly goals, they can stay, either as an in-patient or out-patient, as long as required. When progress in most parameters has tended to plateau, discharge becomes necessary even though ongoing therapy, either physical or psychological, might produce further functional gains. We are aware that our relatively early discharge is not ideal. However, it is usually at this time that locally based therapy becomes more relevant and the role of a regional unit becomes less obvious. The demands upon us are largely due to the virtual non-existence of local rehabilitation teams, that can continue rehabilitation in the longer term.

We see discharged clients either at a formal clinic or alternatively one afternoon per month at a 'drop-in' clinic. At this time any ex-patient or family member may attend and see either the key worker or other specific therapists as desired. This is a useful system and is not dominated by the more demanding individuals. Patients can be re-referred for further periods of in-patient or out-patient rehabilitation, if appropriate, either by themselves or by local therapists or GPs. However, re-referrals are only accepted if a specific purpose and goal can be identified.

LIAISON WITH OTHER REGIONAL SERVICES

We have strong links with the Dene Centre, which is a voluntary organization that houses a regional information service, disabled living centre, continence advisory service and has the NHS Communication Aids Centre within the building. There are also links to the Disablement Services Centre, which acts as a wheelchair prescription service as well as having expertise in prosthetics. There is access to the regional technical aids service, which has bioengineering expertise.

SPECIAL SERVICES AND CLINICS

There has recently been a trend within our unit to develop specialist programmes. Many of these programmes allow group work. Also the, albeit limited, development of local rehabilitation teams has made us concentrate more on highly specialist rehabilitation, which can rarely be undertaken at a local level. All of these services are relevant for discussion in the context of head injury.

Driving

There is a separate driving assessment centre at Hunters Moor. This is run by a senior physiotherapist and a part-time driving instructor with secretarial and medical support. The unit offers assessment and advice with regard to ability to drive as well as advice on adaptations. There are three cars with a variety of adaptations and the vehicles can be used either on a test track within the hospital grounds or on the open road if the client has a valid licence. This is an open referral service and thus not entirely restricted to clients from the regional rehabilitation centre. We find it is a very useful service in that car driving is a vital social activity and much of the later stage rehabilitation process can be usefully carried out in the context of real-life driving situations.

Seating clinic

There is a weekly seating clinic with input from a visiting seating physiotherapist and private orthotist. This is a specialist service for people with more complicated disabilities, who require special seating such as multi-adjustable wheelchairs, Matrix seating, moulded seating, etc. available only for clients who pass through the rehabilitation centre.

Spasticity clinic

This is a specific interest at the hospital and involves a physiotherapist and doctor. The clinic uses a variety of techniques, including serial casting and peripheral nerve blocks with phenol. Such expertise is useful to develop in the context of severe head injury.

Dysarthria programme

This is run by our speech therapists and involves group activity for people with severe dysarthria. It is the subject of a research evaluation at the present time.

Independent living programme

This is run by occupational therapists in conjunction with other members of the rehabilitation team. It started in a very small way with group activity lasting 6 weeks and is often carried out in the bungalows within the hospital grounds, as well as involving a variety of trips into the local community and beyond. Obviously, this is very useful in the context of longer-term community reintegration from head injury and is a service that should be developed. Unfortunately, it is an example of a service that is not clearly the responsibility of a health authority nor of a local authority, and funding for this and other 'tertiary' rehabilitation services is not clear nor readily available at the present time.

Memory programme

Clinical neuropsychology staff run a specific retraining programme for people with memory problems. Once again, this is of major relevance to people with head injury, but requires additional resources and is a programme that is also not clearly the responsibility of a single agency and thus not readily funded.

CONCLUSION

WHAT IS RIGHT WITH OUR SERVICE?

The major advantage of Hunters Moor is that it exists. The hospital now acts as a base for a regional rehabilitation service, with a throughput of approximately 200 clients per annum. It has developed a specific expertise in a number of areas, including the management of people with complex head injury, which in turn includes behavioural disturbance. Such a service was badly needed and has relieved inappropriate pressure on neurosurgical beds, as well as providing access for other patients from around the region. The centre is beginning to provide a focus for education, training and research. It hosts a series of conferences and study days on specific disability topics. Such education and research is vital to the future of rehabilitation. Many of the ways of working described in this chapter are not proved to be better than other methods reviewed in other chapters of this book. Such comparative studies of service delivery are generally not available and are urgently required.

WHAT IS WRONG WITH OUR SERVICE?

The main drawback of the centre is that it is, because of demands upon it, having to concentrate on postacute rehabilitation. We believe this serves a purpose and produces real functional gains for the patient and family and enables people to return home better informed, more ready to cope with an often difficult home situation and, hopefully, in a better physical and emotional state [12,13]. However, it could be argued that many real problems following head injury occur in much later stages, many months and years after the injury. The regional unit cannot adequately deal with these problems, either on geographical grounds or with regard to the potential number of clients involved. The regional centre cannot be all things to all people and should certainly not substitute for the development of good-quality local rehabilitation services. Liaison between ourselves and local teams has been difficult and patchy, and we have sometimes found that patients have physically, cognitively and emotionally declined when we see them a few months later. Regional centres can build up expectations that cannot be fulfilled in the long term and may even rehabilitate to a falsely high level that cannot be reproduced within the home environment. Despite relatively good therapy levels, most patients have many hours in the day unfilled, and an activity organizer would be useful so that structured leisure activities can be pursued within the rehabilitation context. We should involve the family in these activities more than we do and also involve the family in the rehabilitation process in general. The family often needs as much support and counselling as the patient. The unit has not been able to secure good liaison with the vocational rehabilitation service. In the UK, employment rehabilitation is the responsibility of a different Government department, but this should not preclude greater involvement of employment rehabilitationists in the health setting.

SUMMARY

This chapter has outlined the development of a regional rehabilitation service, both in theory and in practice. A regional head injury rehabilitation centre is necessary, but should not be seen as a substitute for the proper and parallel development of locally based services.

REFERENCES

1. Medical Disability Society. *The Management of Traumatic Brain Injury*. London: Development Trust for the Young Disabled, 1988.
2. Cope DN, Hall KA. Head injury rehabilitation: benefits of early intervention. *Archives of Physical Medicine and Rehabilitation* 1982; **63**: 433–437.
3. Wade DT, Langton-Hewer R, Skilbeck CE, David RM. *Stroke – A Critical Approach to Diagnosis, Treatment and Management*. London: Chapman & Hall, 1985.
4. Royal College of Physicians of London. *Physical Disability in 1986 and Beyond*. London: Royal College of Physicians, 1986.
5. Oddy M, Bonham E, McMillan T *et al*. A comprehensive service for the rehabilitation and long-term care of head injury survivors. *Clinical Rehabilitation* 1989; **3**: 253–259.
6. British Psychological Society Working Party. *Services for Young Adult Patients with Acquired Brain Damage*. Leicester: British Psychological Society, 1989.
7. Wade DT. Designing disability services – the Oxford experience. *Clinical Rehabilitation* 1990; **4**: 147–158.
8. West Midlands Regional Health Authority. *A Rehabilitation Service for the West Midlands*. Birmingham: West Midlands Regional Health Authority, 1987.

9. Northern Regional Health Authority Advisory Committee on Disability. *Services for People with a Physical Disability in the Northern Region*. Newcastle upon Tyne: Northern Regional Health Authority, 1989.
10. Pentland B, Barnes MP. Staffing provision for early head injury rehabilitation. *Clinical Rehabilitation* 1988; **2**: 309–313.
11. Eames P, Wood R. Rehabilitation after severe brain injury: a follow-up study of a behaviour modification approach. *Journal of Neurology, Neurosurgery, and Psychiatry* 1985; **48**: 613–619.
12. Cope DN, Cole JR, Hall KM, Barkan H. Brain injury: An analysis of outcome in a post acute rehabilitation system. Part 1: General analysis. *Brain Injury*, 1991; **5**: 111–125.
13. Brooks N. The effectiveness of post acute rehabilitation. *Brain Injury* 1991; **5**: 103–109.

A rural service:
developing rehabilitation in the community

5

Chris Evans

INTRODUCTION

For centuries patients have survived traumatic brain injuries (TBI). Little change has happened in their management until recently. Even now there are few places which have clear strategies, adequate space and staffing during the hospital phase, as well as competent community follow-up and rehabilitation.

DEFINITIONS

The Medical Disability Society (MDS), now renamed the British Society for Rehabilitation Medicine (BSRM), commissioned a working party to produce a report on managing traumatic brain injury. This report was published in 1988. Many of the definitions in this chapter are from that monograph [1]. Most others are from the World Health Organization [2].

WHO GETS TBI?

Field's [3] report identified twin peaks of incidence of head injury – those between the ages of 15 and 19 and those over 75. He confirmed that men are more at risk than women, though when the second peak is reached the difference has all but disappeared. Kraus [4] also demonstrated this. Wade and Langton Hewer [5] and the MDS report reached similar conclusions. Evans [6] reported on the cohort of patients examined from Chessington. In this selected group there was a bias towards the younger age range.

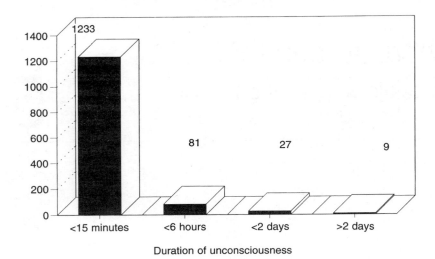

Figure 5.1 Estimated incidence of TBI for population of 450 000 (managed population of Cornwall).

Cornwall, the most south-westerly county in the UK, has a managed population of 450 000. In 1992 there were about 1000 patients discharged from Cornish hospitals with the diagnosis of head injury, approximately 15 of whom were admitted to the Cornwall Stroke and Rehabilitation Unit (CSRU) with very severe TBI. The figures are consistent with those predicted for the very severe group (Figure 5.1).

Until recently, minor, moderate and severe injuries did not appear in the Cornish figures, but a research programme initiated by the Department of Health is investigating this deficiency as part of the National Traumatic Brain Injury Research Study. Since February 1993, all patients who have suffered a head injury and been sent to hospital are being identified, interviewed and followed up. This will give an accurate record of incidence of TBI and also assess the minor brain injury which may follow. The study is expected to last 5 years.

We expect to admit 15–20 patients with severe or very severe TBI annually to the CSRU. It would be difficult to justify a unit for them alone, but it has proved practical to link the management of TBI with younger patients with cerebrovascular accident (CVA), subarachnoid haemorrhage or other intracranial insult. The therapy disciplines required are common, as are many of the problems. This makes it possible to maintain a specialist facility at district level for a rural area.

This is important, because, as argued by Evans and Skidmore [7], a unit geographically remote from the patients' home is only of value in

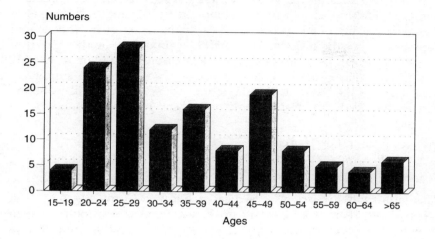

Figure 5.2 TBI survivors presenting for the first time. All had severe or very severe head injuries.

the short term. If it is hoped the patient will go home and be looked after in the community, then maintaining close contact with family and friends is essential. In more populated areas a specialized unit drawing from a population of 1–2 million could be viable.

The expectation of life after surviving the original TBI has been recorded in United States veterans, by Corkin, Sullivan and Carr [8]. They confirm a nearly normal life expectancy, unless epilepsy has supervened. Figure 5.2 shows numbers and ages of survivors of very severe TBI in the County seen by the Rehabilitation Service in Cornwall in the last 9 years.

This shows the expected higher incidence in youth, but a significant number of survivors in later life. This information suggests that facilities for patients with TBI must cover all age groups.

PROCESSES OF REHABILITATION

Processes are to do with technique rather than timing. There are three. The first is the initial rehabilitation process, when an attempt is made to improve patients' abilities as much as possible by whatever means available. This could include remedial therapies, medication and corrective surgery.

The second is to do with reducing handicap by altering the environment when the remaining problems of patients cannot be improved. This process includes adapting housing, transport, clothing.

Finally, the third process is to alter and improve 'behaviour'. Memory, concentration and socializing are embraced by this rather diffuse term 'behaviour'. Part of the process is to help patients, their families and carers to accept the residual and unbidden problems, be they physical or psychological. Part is a wider role to educate the public to tolerate disabled citizens better. All three processes can take place simultaneously, but it is likely that adaptation of behaviour will continue throughout all the phases of rehabilitation and into the community.

PHASES OF REHABILITATION

Acute

This lasts from admission to medical stability. In Cornwall, as in most other places, there is an element of chance about which route is taken through the acute service. Clinical management may be from general surgeons, orthopaedic surgeons, anaesthetists or neurosurgeons. It is not usually a matter of choice, but more a matter of local expediency and practice. The wise patient will take care both where and when to have the head injury. (The wiser still would avoid it altogether!) It might be a little far-fetched to include the emergency services as part of the rehabilitation team, but the end results will be strongly influenced by the way in which patients are managed at the roadside and on the way into hospital.

Postacute

This starts when it becomes clear the patient will survive off ventilation and intubation. Probably the least satisfactory solution is for the patient to be an unwanted guest in a surgical or neurosurgical ward. Acute wards cost more than rehabilitation wards, so it is a costly option. Even minimally disruptive behaviour is intolerable on such a ward and it may lead to inappropriate and potentially damaging sedation being given.

In Cornwall patients are usually sent from intensive treatment unit, surgical ward or the neurosurgical unit direct to the CSRU. The CSRU takes patients who are still unconscious, but they must be detached from ventilator, monitors and intra-arterial lines. Tracheotomies, nasogastric tubes or urinary catheters are not a bar to admission.

This may be the first time that the full impact of the injury becomes apparent to both patient and relatives. After the profound shock that the injury happened, there is almost a heady euphoria in relatives when the patient survives. There is often initial encouragement from visible progress early on, but as the weeks pass progress slows. As the time to leave hospital approaches, it may be clear that the patient's disabilities are going to change the family's way of life for ever. It is usually at this stage that the system fails, because the options are so limited. Brooks has graphically described the impact of TBI on the family [9].

Transition from hospital to home

Even for patients with severe TBI, the time in hospital or other in-patient stay is not usually going to exceed a year. Since most units have no access to a rehabilitation facility, it will mean the choices on leaving hospital are very limited – and that most patients will go home. If there is no community rehabilitation (as is usual), then any progress after discharge will depend on the unskilled and unsupported efforts of the carers. Links between hospital and home are often inadequate and planning for discharge undeveloped. There have been cases where the patient is abruptly sent home to relatives, who have not received instruction, support or even warning. Patients may be placed in residential or nursing home care without the consent of either the relatives or the patient (who sometimes is thought to be in no position to express an opinion).

Such solutions are inappropriate, inconsistent with the Patients' Charter and in some cases illegal. It is at this time that community rehabilitation systems are needed.

Rehabilitation in the community

The ideal outcome after TBI occurs where the patient leaves hospital and, after a period of rehabilitation, takes up his or her original job, has the same income and prospects, lives in the same house as his intact family, is independent of any other person or piece of equipment and enjoys all previous hobbies and social contact. When reality falls short of the ideal, it means that all aspects of quality of life are impaired. The rehabilitation process aims to allow as close a restoration to the original situation as possible. The least satisfactory outcome is where the patient has to be admitted into long-stay care against his/her will, or at least without his/her consent. This may happen for a variety of reasons. There may be nobody in the family to care for the patient at home, or the physical or psychological consequences of the accident may alienate potential carers so much that they are unwilling to have the patient home. Conflict may happen when the patient states a preference to be at home but does not have the insight that his behaviour is stressful, even intolerable.

CONSIDER A HYPOTHETICAL CASE

A young man has been injured in a motor cycle accident. He survived TBI and was unconscious for 2 weeks. He has had global damage. Before the accident he was finishing an apprenticeship. His hobbies were his bike, going to the pub and going out with his girlfriend, with whom he shared a flat. She has gone off the scene now, because she says he is 'not the person she knew'. His parents are in their early 50s and work. Now, 1 year after the accident, he is due to go home. He is unable to concentrate properly and his memory for recent events is flawed. He needs help dressing and in self-care. He walks slowly and unsteadily; speech, the content of which is reasonable, is slow and difficult to understand. He is continent provided someone can take him to the toilet quickly. He is easily frustrated and angry, gets abusive and may be verbally aggressive. There have been fits, and he takes anticonvulsants if he remembers. The fits have stopped him driving. He smokes cigarettes, but forgets where he has left them. He can not be left on his own in the house, for that reason if no other.

He has therefore, lost his job, his girlfriend and his home. He is sufficiently aware to realize that he does not function well, but does not have full insight or memory. The plan being made for him is that he should go back to his parents' home. It is expected that he will qualify for most of the grants and allowances. Adaptations can be made to the house, which will make it accessible. It means that his parents will have to give up work and they are not keen to do this. He does not like the plan. He would like simply to go back to the old flat he had with his girlfriend and cannot see why this is impossible. As second best, he would accept another flat and says he could manage on his own if he had to.

The hospital stay allowed a lot of procrastination. It was only when discharge was imminent that problems that should have been addressed early on were seen for the first time and the services, both in hospital and community, examined the options. They discovered a local residential unit, but the age group was wrong, so he could not be admitted there, even if he liked it (which he did not). They looked for suitably adapted accommodation for him, but they could not find enough money to pay for the full-time carers needed. The multiplicity of problems called for new solutions. Examination of the problems generated by this hypothetical, but credible case helps to define the needs of rehabilitation services for the TBI in the community. He was stuck.

QUESTIONS RAISED BY THE HYPOTHETICAL HISTORY

A role for case managers?

Case managers are extensively used in the United States, and their role is to try to take the overall view of the rehabilitation programmes for many groups of patients, particularly those with TBI. They are enthusiastically supported in the USA by insurance companies, who wish to make it as easy as possible to provide rehabilitation early, since it has been shown to reduce long-term morbidity (and also costs). In the UK the concept of case managers started in a London teaching hospital, where liaison had to be made with many local authorities, social services departments and community services. A therapist was appointed to act as a case manager for the entire rehabilitation process, with the aim of speeding up and improving communications between departments for the patient's benefit.

Ideally, the case manager is introduced to the patient and his family while the patient is on the intensive treatment unit and follows the patient through the hospital system out into the community. Contact will continue as long as it is helpful. This concept will be most important in the long-term community management of patients. There will be an element of advocacy in the job, the case manager being responsible to the patient. It is unfortunate that in the UK, under the new 'care in the community' legislation, some areas have called a tier of officials 'Care Managers' or 'Case Coordinators'. It may lead to confusion as the social services roles are different. They will have access to budgets, so cannot act as advocates in the same way as independent case managers. In this chapter the latter definition is used.

In Cornwall this task has been undertaken for the last 3 years by an occupational therapist who has a shared commitment to the Rehabilitation Unit and the community. It is she who follows the patient from ITU to CSRU, follows up after discharge and, when possible, integrates return to work. In 1993 a second occupational therapist was appointed to share the load. Significantly, both were initially funded by charities. The case manager does not have to be an occupational therapist. Other remedial professions undertake the role. In hospital at least, it could be undertaken by the doctor. Usually it is the lack of time which stops a doctor being the case manager in the sense under discussion. Having an effective case manager will not remove clinical responsibility from the doctor, but may facilitate a more cohesive team.

The role of the general practitioner in the management of the rehabilitation of the head-injured patient will depend on the type of practice. Very few general practitioners have experience or training in rehabilitation. A case manager (in the national sense) could be the ideal point of contact. Some practices are well used to the idea of multi-disciplinary assessment and management. For others it would come as a culture shock of seismic proportions.

Is there freedom to choose by the patient?

In theory, patients have the right to decide where they want to live, with whom and under what conditions. They should be able to take responsibility for their finances and be autonomous. In the UK, the only lawful exceptions are where an Order has been placed on them under the Mental Health Act or if they are in legal custody. In practice there will be compromises, and many decisions are taken on the patient's behalf by relatives and professionals. It is rare for any protection to be given to the patient legally, as a Court of Protection is expensive and will only deal with finance; guardianship is cumbersome. Similarly, giving a Power of Attorney to friends or relatives is most difficult in those very cases where it is needed most, i.e. those whose ability to manage their own affairs is so impaired that their views are not accessible.

Often, patients are as in the hypothetical case, i.e. they can make decisions but no-one feels confident that they will be sufficiently sound. There is another ethical and legal minefield here. Recently the British Medical Association has agreed to the principle of the 'living will', so that in future an individual will be able to give an opinion on the future on a 'what if?' basis and give clear instructions about what they would like to happen.

Network [10], the Living Options partnership journal, describe some instances where it is the patient who is funded, and the patient then employs as much help as is needed, buying the right aids and necessary equipment. Such provision constitutes a true needs-led service, but is very unusual. Living Options is supported by the Kings Fund.

What was the patient like before the injury?

In the hypothetical case the patient had been in stable employment and relationship, with high expectations before the injury. It is not always so. Patients who suffer injury may come from specific sections of the population, even allowing for the already discussed age and sex differentials. It seems common sense that people who are aggressive are more likely to be involved in fights and accidents. Alcohol is thought to be a major factor. Information from the Road Research Laboratory confirms this.

In the Chessington study, time and care was taken to find out what the patient was like before the accident. If, before the accident, the patient was known to be a short-tempered, aggressive boor, or a work-shy, alcoholic layabout, then the occurrence of severe head injury was unlikely to improve his personality. This could not always be assumed, since one aggressive young man was received home by his relatives with glee, for they found him less aggressive than before the accident. In general, it seemed that behaviour and motivation of a patient before the accident had an important bearing on his rehabilitation. Since some of these patients have no family support and poor home environment, they often present the biggest challenge.

Funding and insurance

Only when the patient has comprehensive insurance and was the innocent party in an accident, suffered an industrial injury or was the innocent victim of an assault is there a possibility of help of independent funding. The sources would be the insurance company, if the problem was an attributable accident, or the Criminal Injuries Compensation Board. If it is available, then options extend dramatically. They may include buying suitable residential care in a specialized unit at a distance or adapting and staffing the patient's own home, buying in necessary staff for home care and rehabilitation. Unfortunately, only about 10% of patients with TBI are in a position to make a claim and at present settlements are greatly delayed, rarely being completed until at least 5 years after the accident. Interim payments can be made, but they need to be fought for!

Structured settlements are being used more frequently and have more flexibility. When carefully set up they can secure the future of the patient in any eventuality. Relatives should be advised to instruct a solicitor specializing in these claims as early as possible after the accident. At present, such a course seems the only way to guarantee a full choice, even if it is only for the small minority. If the UK follows the US pattern, they may be used more in the future. In any event, the Case Manager or other responsible professional should ensure that the possibility of interim payments is thoroughly explored.

REHABILITATION IN THE COMMUNITY

In developing facilities for the rehabilitation of TBI in the community, there are some key requirements (Table 5.1).

Such requirements should consist of national, regional and local policies. The manager of a community rehabilitation service need not be a doctor, but must be knowledgeable and enthusiastic and able to manage such a service. However, in the UK it is difficult to get sufficient medical political clout unless the group is represented on local working parties by a consultant.

Table 5.1 Developing teams – some requirements

- Planning groups should include carers and patients
- Manager (might be medical but does not have to be)
- Enthusiast (ditto)
- Rehabilitation teams, vertical and longitudinal
- Resource/mobility centre
- Clear finance (HA, FHSA, SSD, structured settlement)
- Carer and crisis relief centres
- Lifelong monitoring – not by the provider!

PRIMARY HEALTH CARE TEAMS

In the UK, there is already a well-established system of primary care to deal with most medical conditions in the community. It consists of the long-established teams of general practitioners and community nurses, together with their ancillary workers. Community nurses, used to visiting patients in their homes, give much support for specific problems which arise after TBI. However, the links of the primary health care teams with other disciplines needed for managing TBI are poor.

There are too few physiotherapists, occupational therapists, speech therapists or clinical psychologists available to treat and supervise the rehabilitation of patients in the community. Management of TBI does not feature in training of GPs, any more than it does for most doctors. Now that fundholding practices (GPs with their own budget) are developing, it is not certain that these new purchasers will be any more aware of the needs of the patient with TBI than in the past. In any event, it is unlikely that there will be much more money with which to buy services. It will remain essential to make the best uses of what is available.

COMMUNITY REHABILITATION TEAMS

In Cornwall these were started in 1985, in order to improve cooperation between the field workers of social services and health authority, so that their work could be used to best effect. Teams evolved when a patient with severe head injury had been discharged into the community without a rehabilitation programme to follow and without a unit in which it could be undertaken. The speech therapist, occupational therapist, physiotherapist and social worker involved in his care began to meet regularly to plan ways to manage the resources available for him [11]. The idea developed, and there are now six community rehabilitation teams in Cornwall co-terminous with the social services boundaries. Teams have recently started in north Cornwall and south Devon (the neighbouring county), which do not function identically, but the purpose is the same. They all link with a residential facility in south Devon.

Teams hold meetings monthly. Up to about 10 clients may be discussed. Some have been newly referred and others are reviews. In every case, explicit consent has been given for referral and for information to be shared between the social services and health authority staff. It does not matter where the meetings are held, and in practice some are in hospital buildings and others in social services units. It has become usual for the hosting organization to provide the secretarial support. There is a convener of each team, who sends out minutes and agenda, and is responsible for chairing the meeting. Over the years each team has built up considerable knowledge about the local facilities and who needs them.

The health authority representatives include nursing staff from the community, medical staff from the hospitals and therapists from either group. Sometimes it is possible for general practitioners to attend, but this is often difficult. Social services are represented by their occupational therapists, social workers and home care attendants. Officers from the housing, education and other Council departments attend as necessary and so do the Disablement Resettlement Officer and clinical psychologist (Table 5.2).

Table 5.2 Community rehabilitation teams – members

Health authority	Social services
Medical specialist	Social workers
Hospital therapists	Domiciliary occupational therapists
Community therapists	Home care organizer
Community nurses	
As needed:	
GPs – if possible	Disablement Resettlement Officer
	Housing Officer

Members recognize that time spent in these meetings saves much time on the telephone and writing letters. Such meetings make response to the patient's problems quicker, reduce bureaucracy and minimize time-wasting.

For most patients who survive TBI the later rehabilitation could, and should, be done at home. Even the medical input traditionally given in out-patients could probably be more effectively provided in the patient's home by the specialist visiting.

OTHER HOME SERVICES

Physiotherapy is available at home in some areas of Cornwall. For most patients with CVA or TBI the service comes from Physiotherapy at Home (PatH), but one or two local hospital are developing a domiciliary service. PatH is charity funded. The social services provide a range of domiciliary services which include occupational therapy. A recent new post in the CSRU will provide speech therapy and is intended to be between the unit and home. The second occupational therapist and the art therapist appointed in the last few months are also funded by a charity.

Art therapy is a discipline rarely found in rehabilitation teams. The therapist works mostly on the unit but, as with the other members of the team, follows up appropriate patients after discharge. The central concern of the art therapist is the emotional wellbeing of the patient. Common themes explored are loss, anger, frustration, lack of confidence and problems in coping with leaving the Unit. The non-verbal nature of art therapy reaches out to otherwise inaccessible patients.

HELP IN RETURNING TO WORK

A retrospective survey, funded by the Nuffield Provincial Hospitals Trust, is looking at all patients seen by the service over the last 10 years. This is already helping to identify gaps in services more accurately. We are recording the outcome of past rehabilitation methods. One of the outcome measures is employability. Even in Cornwall, which is an area of high unemployment, the study already shows that a significant percentage of patients who have been through the Unit in the last 10 years have managed to get back to work, some against the odds.

Recent legislation has removed the Disablement Resettlement Officer and most of the employment centres have gone. They have been replaced by Disability Employment Advisers (DEA), and in each area there is a PACT (Placement Assessment and Counselling Team). There will also be a Committee for the Employment of People with Disability (CEPD). As there is significant unemployment locally amongst the whole population as well as those with TBI, in practical terms, unless there is good recovery and an enlightened employer, return to work is difficult.

On a more positive note, a recent initiative from the EEC social fund allows the use of open learning centres by physically handicapped patients with TBI for rehabilitation. It will make it possible to attend conventional training establishments and be part of the link into work experience and training schemes.

ASSESSMENTS AND AUDIT

Any changes made need to be seen to be effective. Therefore, accurate measurement of both the activity and the outcome is essential. While accurate assessments are invaluable, many assessments are often merely displacement activities for staff; they produce no valid information since no useful question was asked; and they are done to give the illusion of activity. If time used in assessment is to be well spent, then they need to be well-designed and relevant, repeatable, recordable and retrievable [12].

Over the last 3 years, assessments of dependency have been developed in Cornwall as part of the rehabilitation package for the South Western RHA Medical Data Index system. This is based on the patient administration system, which already controls appointments, admissions and record tracing. It is used to provide the demographic data of each patient who comes into hospital. The information about the specific episode of illness is added, together with an assessment of handicap, which can be upgraded each week while on the ward and at any subsequent contact [13].

THE FUTURE

Until quite recently, it was believed that recovery from head injury took place during the first few months only. Any improvement observed later was assumed to be due to adaptation, not neurological improvement. This view is now changing, and observations of workers over recent years suggest that neurological recovery continues for longer than 6 months. In a conference in Bordeaux in April 1991 many issues were examined in detail [14]. Speakers emphasized the underlying flexibility of the central nervous system to change, and this approach to the neurophysiology of recovery gives encouragement and challenge to those whose work is mainly concerned with neurological rehabilitation. The recognition of the plasticity of the nervous system, the presence of unused pathways capable of retraining and the recognition of the complexity of the synaptic system around the anterior horn cell give us encouragement; they suggest that there may be a neurophysiological basis for recovery which is far better than mere adaptation.

Mechanisms of recovery are becoming clearer [15], but it has yet to be proved that an intensive rehabilitation programme, involving all disciplines intensively, can be justified in terms of its effectiveness. Methods of delivery, such as therapies in the community, need to be worked out. The fact that 50% of the young men intensively treated in the Joint Services Rehabilitation Unit at Chessington returned to work, compared with the 15% in the MDS survey, suggests that the current situation could be improved.

Controlled studies of rehabilitation are difficult to design and execute. Knowledge may be more successfully gained by repeated careful case studies. A review by Wagenaar and Meijer in 1990 [16], looking at 165 studies on the effectiveness of rehabilitation, showed that patients benefit from expert care and suggested that the early start of intensive treatment seems important. It seemed that the generalization to ADL from specific exercises was not convincing, although visual perception training showed benefit which could be transferred to reading and writing. There remains a major problem of how to develop improvements in ADL skills.

This extract from the last paragraph of a chapter was written 10 years ago, but it serves as well today as then:

The challenge consists to establish that an intensive rehabilitation programme involving periods of physiotherapy, occupational therapy and speech therapy throughout the day for several days a week can be justified in terms of effectiveness. It is also necessary to establish whether one particular method of rehabilitation is better than another. There are many systems, which have been devised, and claims are made for each but there are no figures with which to support these arguments. This lack is due to the one fundamental deficiency in rehabilitation and that is of accurate measurements. Until these are available there is no scientific foundation for the belief that rehabilitation works. Inwardly, one may have the conviction that it does, but in the future, with increasing competition for funds, conviction alone will be inadequate.

REFERENCES

1. McLellan D *et al. The Management of Traumatic Brain Injury.* London: The Development Trust for the Young Disabled, Medical Disability Society, c/o Royal College of Physicians, 1988.
2. World Health Organization. *International Classification of Impairments, Disabilities and Handicaps (ICIDH) in Rehabilitation.* Strasbourg: Council of Europe Publications and Documents Division, 1989.
3. Field JH. *A Study of the Epidemiology of Head Injury in England and Wales, with Particular Reference to Rehabilitation (A Report to the DHSS).* London: Department of Health and Social Security, 1975.
4. Kraus JF *et al.* The incidence of acute brain injury with severe impairment in a defined population. *American Journal of Epidemiology,* 1984; **119**: 186–891.
5. Wade D, Langton-Hewer R. Epidemiology of some neurological conditions with specific reference to the workload on the NHS. *International Rehabilitation Medicine* 1987; **8**: 129–137.
6. Evans CD. Long term follow-up of head injured patients. In: Eames P, Wood RL, eds. *Models of Brain Injury Rehabilitation.* London: Academic Press, 1989.
7. Evans CD. Long-term follow-up of head injuries. In: Eames P, Wood RL, eds. *Models of Brain Injury Rehabilitation.* London: Chapman & Hall, 1991: pp 184–203.
8. Corkin S, Sullivan E, Carr A. Prognostic factors of life expectancy after penetrating head injury. *Archives of Neurology* 1977; **41**: 975.
9. Brooks DN, Campsie LM, Symington C *et al.* The five year outcome of severe blunt head injury: a relative's view. *Journal of Neurology, Neurosurgery, and Psychiatry* 1986; **49**: 764–770.
10. *Network* (Journal of the Living Options Partnership) can be obtained from the King's Fund Centre, 126 Albert Street, London, NW1 7NF.
11. Evans CD. Community rehabilitation. *Clinical Rehabilitation* 1987; **1**: 133–137.
12. Evans CD. Rehabilitation of brain injury. In: Illis L, ed. *Neurological Rehabilitation,* 2nd ed. Oxford: Blackwell Scientific Publications, 1993.
13. Evans CD, Gibson J, Jones T, Williams M. A medical diagnostic index for rehabilitation. Disability and Rehabilitation, 1993; 15(3): 127–135.
14. Pélissier J, Barat M, Mazaux JM. Traumatismé Cranien grave et Médecine de Rééducation, Masson, Paris, 1991.

15. Bach-y-Rita P. Biological and psychosocial factors in the recovery from brain damage in humans. Canadian Journal of Psychology, 1990; 44: 148–165.
16. Wagenaar RC, Meijer OG. Effects of stroke rehabilitation (1). Journal of Rehabilitation Sciences, 1991; 4: 61–70.

An urban community service:

head injury – using occupational therapy to meet the challenge of community reintegration

6

David Hughes, Elizabeth Ward, Heather Warnock, Ruth Hunter, Alan Tennant and M. Anne Chamberlain

INTRODUCTION AND EARLY DEVELOPMENTS

Murphy and colleagues [1] provided evidence to suggest that in the UK the current services available to those who have sustained a head injury, are inadequate and often inappropriate. Nationally, as Cockburn and Gatherer [2] showed, there are wide regional differences in the availability of rehabilitation. In a review of 19 centres that had some in-patient beds occupied by adults who had suffered a head injury they found that specific provision tailored to the rehabilitation needs of adults after head injury appeared to be rare. A recent report from the Royal College of Physicians of London [3] found that there are few resources specifically dedicated to the needs of the head-injured population.

In 1988 a working party was set up in the West Yorkshire area of the UK to examine the needs of patients after a head injury and the response of the health and welfare services to those needs [4]. The report identified that there was little provision of acute in-patient rehabilitation or provision and coordination of services for head-injured patients once discharged from hospital: 'Many patients are lost to follow-up, and patients are often inappropriately placed and managed during the progressing phases of their care.' The link between hospital and community was deemed to be vital and, as a result of the working party, it was decided to try and improve community reintegration following head injury. This led to a project being established in the administrative area of Leeds City Council which shares its boundary with the Leeds Health District. These authorities serve a population of over 710 000 people and the district includes compact urban areas of Leeds city as well as smaller towns such as Wetherby, together with rural areas around the periphery.

In the year ending March 1990, almost 1500 Leeds residents were discharged from hospital following head injury. Overall, the annual incidence rate for admission to hospital following head injury was 211 per 100 000, based on admission for fracture of the skull and intracranial injury but excluding fracture of the facial bones. The young and the old have higher incidence rates and the rate for males is roughly twice that of females. Nearly seven in every eight (86%) were discharged within 2 days.

Rehabilitation in Leeds is well developed and is characterized by a multisite structure, with facilities including two major teaching hospitals, the local authority and the independent sector. Early rehabilitation services are provided on the neurosurgical wards, but those with moderate or severe head injury are often transferred to a national demonstration centre in rehabilitation nearby, providing a neurorehabilitation service. A consultant in rehabilitation works from the General Infirmary and the neurorehabilitation facility, as well as other sites, with a specific brief for head injury. In addition, a community hospital has a Young Disabled Unit, offering day therapy, and a Young Adult Team, a multi-disciplinary team established in 1989 to provide a specialized community rehabilitation service to those aged 16–25 years. A Disabled Living Centre is located on the same site.

By 1990 Leeds City Council Social Services employed 23 community occupational therapists (OT) and 18 OT assistants in the Leeds District. This expanding service implies a level of cover from qualified community OTs of the order of 3.2 per 100 000 people, with a national target for this service of 5.0 per 100 000 people. Services are well developed; there are two resource centres specifically for young people with disabilities, other day-care provision and a range of other help, including specialist social workers for physical disability and for sensory impairment as well as specialist benefit advisors.

This diffuse model of rehabilitation and associated social services is typical of the structure of rehabilitation services throughout Britain, although better developed in the Leeds district than is commonly found in the UK. Nevertheless, the working party report revealed shortfalls which had to be addressed; in particular it recognised the difficulty of organizing and sustaining appropriate services for patients leaving hospital, especially those who did not easily fit into existing community services. Discussions between social services and a University-based team funded by a grant from the Nuffield Provincial Hospitals Trust, a

UK charity working in the field of health care innovation, led to the establishment of a project, which, with respect to those who have had a head injury, sought to: (1) investigate the possibility of effective management of people at home and (b) develop the role of occupational therapy within Leeds City Council as part of their response to the 1986 Disability Act [5], and the then recent Community Care White Paper [6].

It was, therefore, decided to establish a project to:

1. set up a register of patients discharged after head injury, recording those adults who were Leeds residents and those who had spent greater than 24 hours in the neurosurgical unit;

and for those meeting these criteria the aims were:

2. to assess the patient's needs as soon as possible after discharge by a community OT assessment, including some standardized assessment methods and with follow up at least on an annual basis;
3. to coordinate services to maximize the level of independence available;
4. to identify gaps in the service and thus recommend changes to improve the recovery process.

The thrust of the project was to determine how far community reintegration could be brought about by coordinating existing services with some relatively low-cost additional developments, rather than by developing a single dedicated facility. This response is in line with suggestions made by Wade with respect to managing patients who present difficult problems with multiple disabilities following head injury. He argues that: 'The temptation to set up a new service specifically for head-injured patients should be resisted. Instead, existing services should be used. This necessarily includes social services.' [7]

The focus on neurosurgery, which only accounts for some 5% of discharges following head injury, reflects a pragmatic developmental approach to following up those who were most likely to have severe problems with community reintegration. It was thought that experience with this group of patients would help decide upon the resource implications and practicality of following up other patients with head injury.

A coordinator for the project was also appointed. The coordinator's action role is similar to the role of a 'family advocate' [8], i.e.:

1. to identify a high priority service need;
2. to find an existing service delivery system that could be modified to meet the identified need;
3. to provide assistance in the planning and the implementation of appropriate modifications;

4. to help establish an assessment process to ensure that the plan was properly implemented and modified if necessary.

The high priority need had been identified by the working party and the existing service of community occupational therapy was identified as a potential vehicle for responding to that need. OTs were thought to be particularly suitable, because (1) their training encompasses both physical and psychological aspects of rehabilitation and (2) in the UK many local authorities employ OTs to work in the community.

The first steps in planning and implementing modifications to existing services were taken in mid 1989, when the coordinator began working with both the social services community OTs and with the consultants in neurosurgery to establish a database to identify those meeting the criteria for follow-up. At that time there was no experience of audit in neurosurgery, although audit for stroke patients was established in the neurorehabilitation facility. A paper version of the audit was set up for a 3-month period, concentrating on the basic information thought appropriate to traumatic brain injury. Thus, the Glasgow Coma Score [9] and duration of (1) coma and (2) post-traumatic amnesia were recorded, as were diagnostic and intervention data, the type of discharge and the Glasgow Outcome Scale (GOS) [10].

The audit was established on the neurosurgery department's computer from January 1990 and 156 patients who were admitted to neurosurgery during that year were recorded on the audit. Adding five long-stay patients carried over from 1989, the average age of the 161 patients treated during 1990 was 31.1 years (median 23 years). The average length of stay was 39.2 days (median 7 days). As this suggests, the data were highly skewed by the long-stay patients. The average length of stay for those patients admitted during 1990 was 15.8 days (median 7 days). The Glasgow Coma Scale of patients on admission showed an average score of 8.2 (median 8).

Half (51%) of those treated during 1990 made a 'good recovery', according to the Glasgow Outcome Scale. Just over one in five (21%) died; nearly one-fifth (18%) were discharged with moderate disability and 4% of patients treated were discharged with severe disability. Thus, almost a quarter of patients admitted were discharged with moderate or severe disability, but only one in five of these were transferred to the specialized neurorehabilitation ward for, as with most other places, head-injured persons had to compete with other patients, such as those who had had a stroke, for scarce rehabilitation resources.

Having developed the database to provide a better understanding of potential demand and to be able to refer those adult residents who had stayed for longer than a day (which initially would pick up many who had made a 'good recovery'), how were the community OTs going to respond? The Social Services community OTs already responded to 250 new referrals every week, an annual demand of about 18 per 1000 residents, mostly for assistive devices to maintain independence of the elderly. With an average of 12 new referrals each week for each OT, the scope for taking on clients who had the potential for presenting a wide range of problems and needs, and particularly those beyond the normal range of intervention determined largely by prescriptive legislation, was severely limited. The challenge lay in determining how far the OTs were able to provide the comprehensive assessment and possibly treatment to those with a head injury, as well as some support to the family.

Initially, three community OTs (one from each of the new divisions covering Leeds that were to become operational in April 1990) were designated to respond to head injuries. OT time had to be negotiated with managers and, in the event, each OT was allowed to give a day a week to their head-injured patients. This represents a resourcing level of about one whole-time equivalent OT for one million people, responding to adults discharged from neurosurgery following head injury.

The first task OTs faced was to develop a comprehensive system of assessment for the head-injured person and their family. The 'handicap' dimensions of the International Classification of Impairments, Disabilities and Handicaps (ICIDH) [11], shown in Table 6.1, were used as guidelines for the areas that needed to be assessed.

Table 6.1   The International Classification of Impairments Disabilities and Handicaps – handicap scales

1.	Orientation
2.	Physical independence
3.	Mobility
4.	Occupation
5.	Social integration
6.	Economic self-sufficiency

The assessment instrument was developed incrementally, with measures added and discarded as experience suggested they were unsuitable. Standardized measures were used wherever possible, and included a 'modified Barthel' assessment [12,13] and a set of summary scales based on the ICIDH handicap dimensions.

In addition, both patients and principal carers were assessed using the Nottingham Health Profile [14,15]. This is a simple self-completed instrument for assessing health status. A functional assessment was undertaken and leisure, social needs, communication, cognition and behaviour were examined. The Short Test of Mental Status [16] was found to offer a useful screen for cognition, but a screen for behaviour was difficult to find and was limited to questioning the patient and, wherever possible, their main carer.

Client and family support services were also listed, including the range of benefits they were receiving. A checklist was devised to identify the range of other services involved.

The time taken and the difficulties encountered in developing and using such an assessment should not be underestimated. The original assessment instrument took about 6 months to develop. OTs in hospital, particularly those in rehabilitation units, may use some standardized measures such as the Rivermead Assessment Battery [17], but there is no tradition of approaching assessment in such a standardized way, either in the hospital or in the community. Furthermore, community OTs have great pressure on their time, and some standardized assessments take considerable time to carry out and score. As such, although use of standardized measures would appear important for an equitable distribution of scarce resources, community OT assessment and practice was individualistic.

The nature of impairments and disabilities arising from head injury led the OTs to broaden the assessment to include aspects such as cognition, occupation and orientation, and to consider appropriate referral for benefits and other needs. In other words, the comprehensive assessment was also shifting OT practice into a wider focus and providing the opportunity to act as a 'key worker' – as a coordinator of services for that particular phase of care, in this instance the immediate post discharge period.

In what way does the role of key worker differ from that of a case manager? Intagliata [18] describes case management as comprising:

1. a comprehensive assessment of individual needs;
2. the development of an individualised package of care to meet those needs;
3. ensuring that the individual gains access to these services;
4. monitoring the quality of services provided and liaising with service providers, if the quality or contents of the services does not meet what is required.

Effectively the community OTs, acting as key workers, were carrying out the first two parts of this programme. Assuring that an individual gained access to a service was dealt with by referral, not by advocacy or other means. Thus the OTs were essentially operating within the resources that were available at the local level. Although they called case conferences with a range of service providers to facilitate provision, the role of advocacy (i.e. a sustained campaign on the client's behalf to gain access to services or other requirements) and long-term management were largely absent. Where long-term involvement was required, then the role of key worker was transferred to another appropriate professional.

Problems were encountered almost immediately. The first major hurdle was that, with their existing workload, the OTs simply could not find the time to carry out the comprehensive assessment they had developed. Managers also found it difficult to adjust to the changes that were required. Fortunately, these problems coincided with a change in policy at the departmental level in responding to referrals, brought about by community care policy developments and the need to target 'risk factors' as a mechanism for rationing service response. A 'priority system' was introduced, effectively giving head-injured patients, as well as other groups like those with malignant disease, the highest priority for response. This priority change gave the community OTs more time to develop their approach to head injury, allowing them to spend a day a week on these cases.

Development time was also enhanced by the appointment of OT assistants to help fully-qualified OTs in their work: it is unlikely that any real advance would have been achieved without this commitment on the part of the social services department.

Knowing the demands being placed on OTs, both in the short-term and while they were undertaking developmental work, it was felt important to monitor the input of OT time as well as identifying the range and type of needs which were being uncovered. This led to the development of the first stage of a community OT audit – a therapy audit to parallel the clinical audit undertaken in neurosurgery. Early results showed that assessments were taking on average 2½ hours. With travel and contact time this meant 50% of total allocated weekly time could be used by assessing one person. In practice, assessments were highly variable, some requiring several visits, others just an hour or so.

OTs also had difficulty in contacting some patients, particularly some of the highly mobile younger males. At an early stage, restrictions had to be placed on the amount of time and effort put into contacting clients. As OTs were spending a considerable amount of time travelling to clients' homes only to find no one at home, those clients with under 5 days stay in hospital were given a limited number of visits, letters or phone calls. In practice, OTs were only able to make contact with about 60% of those discharged. This inability to follow up was to be a serious block on the development of a comprehensive follow-up service for those with head injury. Later, the audit was to confirm that those with less than 5 days stay were relatively free of handicap at follow-up, and by the autumn of 1991 follow-up was restricted to those staying for 5 days or longer.

What about the severity of disability and handicap found in those followed-up? Most patients were found to have mild or moderate injuries making rapid physical recovery, but with varying duration of post-traumatic syndrome. A few had significant physical or communication disorders which were slow to be resolved. Occasionally, there were those with prolonged coma and severe physical deficits, who may continuously or intermittently benefit from rehabilitation over several years [19].

However, for the community OTs, clients also fell into three groups, vis-à-vis the assessment:

- those who had made a good recovery and for whom much of the assessment was inappropriate;
- those for whom the assessment was appropriate;
- those who were in crisis, for whom direct and immediate action was required and for whom the full assessment was too premature.

The inability to follow up some patients was due to the fact that they had returned to work within a week or so and often did not want to be bothered by an assessment. Where this type of patient was seen and assessed, it was generally thought that much of the assessment was inappropriate, covering too much when a quick check would have sufficed. Occasionally, at the other extreme, the OT could not assess because the patient or family was in great distress. For example, in one case the OT's only action was to make an immediate referral to the specialist social worker and to the rehabilitation consultant, as just a week or so after discharge she had found the patient and family unable to cope with the patient's major problems. This is, perhaps, an important reminder of the 'safety-net' value of follow-up in itself, and the fact that the OT was able to refer appropriately, demonstrated her increasing confidence to link into appropriate services, the OT referring in this case directly to the rehabilitation consultant.

This wider 'networking' role was also fostered by an initiative led by social services, who set up a workshop for those working in the field so that resource knowledge could be shared. It was surprising how little those working in the field knew of other resources. As a result, a 'Filofax'-style resource book was produced, with over 100 local and national services that could be utilized to help. However, much the greatest problem has been in adjusting OT practice to be able to offer therapy beyond the confines of that limited by prescriptive legislation. The tradition of responding to physical independence and mobility, and the provision of assistive devices and modifications to the home, itself a specialist service, has proved to be a difficult basis for expansion because of managerial and time constraints placed upon community OTs. For example, offering therapy to improve memory in a community setting is time-consuming, and initially the community OTs appeared to lack the confidence and expertise to offer this kind of treatment.

It became clear that an intensive, sustained training programme was necessary to facilitate this shift in orientation. All the OTs were sent to conferences and workshops on head injury, and local workshops on rehabilitation for memory problems and post traumatic syndrome were organized. In addition, OTs met on a regular basis – on average about half a day a month – with the coordinator and, from mid-1990, with other OTs working with head-injured patients in the health service. It was thought that regular development meetings of this kind were essential to support new initiatives and to make workers feel supported, particularly when much of their work is on an individual basis in people's homes. It soon become clear that the learning and support programme had to be sustained to accommodate staff change. In addition, developing a programme of cognitive rehabilitation requires a level of skill and confidence which can only come by adequate training and by regular application.

RESULTS

CASE HISTORIES

Examples of case histories demonstrating the use of the community OT to promote community reintegration are shown in the boxes. They reflect different levels of involvement on the part of the OT.

Minimum involvement

Clive was a 62-year-old, married building contractor working away from home when he fell 10 feet from scaffolding on to a hard surface. He was admitted to the local hospital, where he was in a coma for almost a day. After 5 days he was transferred to the neurosurgery department at the teaching hospital. Following a further 9 days stay he was discharged home and, shortly after, referred to the community OT.

Prior to his accident, Clive was very fit and worked long hours to help him purchase the house which he had previously rented from his local council. The community OT visited soon after discharge and carried out a comprehensive assessment. With a Barthel [12] score of 95 (out of a possible 100), Clive was managing around the home with only minimal assistance, although he had some restriction in the range of motion of his shoulder. His dizziness restricted his mobility outside the home, so that he preferred to be taken in a car by his son. It was also the major obstacle to returning to work and, in addition, his nearness to retirement age meant that early retirement was a distinct possibility. Clive was anxious about his ability to continue his mortgage payments while on sickness benefit.

The OT's treatment consisted of (1) assessment, (2) referral and (3) giving encouragement to Clive's wife in her purchase of a dog! After assessment the OT referred Clive to the community physiotherapist for further treatment and to the local social services benefits advice worker. The family was also put in touch with the local Headway (The National Head Injuries Association) group as they wanted advice on the most effective way of dealing with a possible compensation claim. The OT also supported Clive's wife in purchasing a dog to help Clive fill in his time and stop him getting in his wife's way, a source of increasing friction. This was the limit of the OT's intervention required in this case, other than (1) letting the family know that she could be contacted if problems arose and (2) a routine 12-month follow-up.

At 12 months Clive was found to be fully independent, although he had not returned to work. The benefits advice worker had sorted out his financial affairs and he had gained further assistance from state benefits. He occupied himself in various ways, including walking his dog, homemaking and childminding his grandchildren. A compensation claim was pending.

Moderate involvement

David was 21 years old when a car left the road and crashed into the wall where he was sitting. He sustained both head and spinal injuries, which led to a stay in neurosurgery and the regional spinal unit. He had a stabilizing rod inserted into his back at the spinal unit from where, after a total of 7 weeks in hospital, he was discharged home doubly incontinent and unable to walk more than a few unsteady steps. Home was with his parents in their three-bedroomed council-owned property. He found great difficulty in attaining independent mobility but, nevertheless, he refused to use the wheelchair outside, preferring to struggle to walk. Initially he would not go outside at all, as he felt people would stare at him. His physical appearance was, and remains, very important to him and he considered that he was trapped within a body that was 'alien'. He relied heavily on his parents for support. Indeed, his father had given up work to care for him.

With his father's help, he set a strict rehabilitation programme for himself which involved weights, walking and exercising on a daily basis. Little professional therapy had been offered, in part due to the fact that he was transferred home from out of the district. A district nurse visited twice weekly but appeared to have made no attempt to mobilize any other resources.

When visited by the community OT some 6 months after discharge (the delay bought about by picking up the out-of-district referral), David presented with a slow, unsteady gait pattern. He had discarded the wheelchair, mobilizing within the home on two elbow crutches. Although he relied on car transport, he could only tolerate a seated position for 10 minutes. He was independent in transfers, did not require help with his catheter and carried out manual evacuation of his bowels. Bathing was difficult due to his unsteadiness. However, his whole focus appeared to be on his programme of exercise, geared to achieving independence.

Following assessment, a range of services was brought together by the OT to achieve a series of short- and longer-term goals that had been negotiated with the patient and his family. Interventions included:

- referral for physiotherapy;
- referral to the recently formed Young Adult Team;
- referral to the benefits advice worker from social services;
- referral to a specialist social worker for people with a physically disability;
- referral to a psychologist.

The OT arranged with the specialist social worker to examine driving potential and carers support groups and with the psychologist where they concentrated on teaching coping strategies to aid socialization. More recently, with the help of the specialist social worker, David has just begun an instructor's course to teach weightlifting to those who have a physical disability. He drives short distances independently but has yet to gain the confidence for longer journeys. Nevertheless, the combined efforts of David, his parents and an extensive package of health and social services input has seen a reasonably successful start to community reintegration, with a better prospect of employment once his training is complete.

Maximum involvement

Edward sustained a head injury, leading to a left-hemiplegia, after being knocked off his bicycle by a lorry. At the time he was 17, studying for A levels which would give him entrance to university, for which he had an offer of a place the following year. Edward had particular interests in computers and would thus spend much time in his own room.

Following his accident, he spent over 6 months in neurosurgery and the local neurorehabilitation facility before being discharged home with a Barthel score of 95. The community OT visited some 5 weeks after discharge. Edward was known to have problems with sequencing as well as left-sided neglect, particularly evident when dressing or walking.

His memory and concentration were impaired and he would often simply walk away from a task without explanation. When in a standing position he had limited weightbearing on the left lower limb. He walked with a rolling gait and he invariably leaned to the left. However, he could mobilize independently on the flat and he was independent in climbing stairs. Nevertheless, his balance was poor and he had developed vertigo. With a left-hemiparesis, he had no useful movement at the wrist or hand.

Following assessment, the OT decided with Edward and his parents what improvements could be made and she arranged a series of interventions. She worked with Edward and his parents to overcome memory problems, including keeping diaries and using activity checklists. Ways in which his parents could help reinforce this therapy were also examined and they tried to get Edward to establish a clear routine to his daily activities. Assistive devices were provided to help improve independence, and a re-referral was made to the rehabilitation consultant so that Edward could spend 5 days in the independent living flat at the local neurorehabilitation facility to assess his safety when performing kitchen tasks. Further equipment to support these new skills was provided upon his return home. Finally, a referral was made to the specialist social worker and to the Young Adult Team, particularly for further physiotherapy.

Just over a year following his first discharge the OT decided to organize a case conference with all those concerned, as progress seemed to have halted and Edward and his parents were complaining that they had lost all sense of direction. Physiotherapy was discontinued at this point as Edward's gait pattern had improved. The Young Adult Team representative, the Disablement Resettlement Officer, the Special Needs Coordinator at the local further education college, the specialist social worker for the physically disabled, the community OT, Edward and his family decided that a short-term plan would be to arrange courses which would reinforce independence skills and that longer-term plans for attending a residential college would be pursued. In the meantime, the local social services resource centre would be approached to help Edward find some voluntary work, and he was referred to the local employment rehabilitation centre for assessment.

These three case studies show how advances have been made with respect to meeting the needs of individual patients and their families. They outline what we now believe to be the parameters for useful and successful intervention under this type of model, having excluded those with a few days stay who return to work very quickly. Clive had relatively simple needs requiring assessment and appropriate referral. David required a more complex response with liaison and networking of resources. Edward required sustained management and treatment, including organising a case conference, liaising with local rehabilitation, social and employment services. This is probably the most complex response under this model of service delivery and provides a useful 'tracer' case in that, if the services can cope well with all Edward's needs, they will probably also respond well to those which are simpler and of shorter duration.

RESEARCH

How far are these examples typical of the new pattern of service being offered to Leeds residents following discharge from neurosurgery? A separate evaluation of the innovation has been carried out to examine the overall efficacy of the project. The background characteristic of those followed up for the research are shown in Tables 6.2 and 6.3, where two groups are identified, those discharged before the new service was fully operational (April 1990) the 'before' group and those discharged after (mostly after October 1990) the 'after' group.

Table 6.2 Background characteristics of those followed up, as a percentage within each group and in total

Characteristic	Before	After	Total
Caused by RTA	47.1	51.9	49.2
Single	55.9	38.5	48.3
Male	73.5	76.9	75.0
Lives alone	17.6	11.5	15.0
Has telephone	88.2	84.6	86.7
Non-manual	25.0	29.2	26.9
A Levels or beyond	21.1	25.0	24.5
Discharged with moderate or severe disability (GOS)	38.2	55.6	45.9
Saw psychiatrist in year before	6.3	11.1	8.5
Number in group	34	27	61

Table 6.3 Background characteristics of those followed up, shown as mean values within each group and in total (GCS = Glasgow Coma Scale score)

Characteristic	Before	After	Total
Average age	35.0	40.5	37.4
Average GCS	9.8	8.1	9.1
Average stay (days)	36.8	34.6	35.8
Average no of cars in household	1.1	0.7	0.9
Average time to follow-up (months)	17.8	12.6	15.5
Number in group	34	27	61

Given the small numbers involved, the most striking fact is the similarities between groups. No single characteristic shows a statistically significant difference between the 'before' and 'after' groups but there are trends, in that those in the 'after' group were more likely to have been in an RTA, were older, in non-manual work with A levels or higher. However, the most important difference must be that they were more likely to be discharged home with moderate or severe disability, but this difference also just failed to reach statistical significance.

If the OTs were making any impact on the care and resulting quality of life of clients, where would we expect to see measurable change? From the case histories given above, we might reasonably expect to find a significant increase in the number of agencies brought to bear on any one case, particularly those offering community-based services. With hindsight we would now expect a better quality of interface between agencies, but we did not measure this aspect. We might also hope to find improvement in various 'quality of life' measures. Follow-up was too soon to assess any differences in return-to-work status of clients, (only 4 months longer than the average time off sick), and the worsening economic situation would make comparison difficult in any case. Our expectations are, therefore, relatively modest – a better 'package of care' and improvement in aspects of quality of life – for example, emotional wellbeing and social isolation – which can be considered important *vis-à-vis* the burden of disability. We would hope that there would be some improvement in the quality of life of carers. Such modest expectations may, nevertheless, prove difficult to quantify.

There is no evidence from Table 6.4 that the 'packages of care', expressed as the number of services involved, have increased in size as a result of the project. The increase in the average number of agencies, either in the community, or in total, can be more than accounted for by the additional presence of the community OT! Weekly numbers of contacts with relatives is higher for the 'after' group, as is the sequelae score.

Table 6.4 Post-injury characteristics of those followed up, shown as mean values within each group and in total

Characteristic	Before	After	Total
Hospital services	1.2	1.3	1.2
Community-based services	1.0	1.5	1.2
All services	2.2	2.7	2.4
Contact with relatives	2.5	4.2	3.3
Sequelae score	66.5	84.5	74.7
Number in group	34	27	61

This 'sequelae score' has been compiled from 42 statements about sequelae following head injury, ranging from headaches, through problems with memory, to destructive behaviour. Respondents are asked to give a score ranging from −10 (infinitely better since injury) to +10 (infinitely worse since head injury). Principal carers are also asked to rate clients on the same scale. The minimum and maximum scores are −420 and +420 respectively, and so the averages shown in Table 16.4 indicate a deterioration in many areas. A key aspect of this scale is that it is rated with respect to the client's judgment about the change in individual sequelae since before the injury. Although there are obvious problems when memory is impaired (when the carer's judgment is taken as proxy), the advantage of this approach over a simple checklist of sequelae is that it accounts for the fact that many head-injured persons displayed behavioural traits previous to their injury. Results from the NHP and the General Health Questionnaire (GHQ) [20] showed no statistical significance (Mann–Whitney) between groups. The percentage of clients having a score equivalent to referral for psychological inter-vention (caseness) on the GHQ was 21.9% for the 'before' group and 25.9% for the 'after' group, which is not significantly different ($p = 0.716$). A quarter of all those followed up had scores above the intervention threshold.

It would seem from these data that univariate techniques fail to identify the merits of the new service described earlier in the case histories. Fortunately, multivariate techniques [21,22] can help us to re-examine the data for potentially more complex relationships. Looking at the level of agencies active with clients in the case histories, given nearly half (48%) of those in the 'before' group had no follow-up at all to their homes, can we predict those who received two or more services to the home following discharge? A logistic regression technique [21] allows us to examine this relationship while controlling for a potential set of confounders, including GOS, age, sex, living in a family or not and time to follow-up. The resulting (main effects) model tells us that, for each day spent in hospital, the odds of receiving two or more services following discharge are raised by 1.02 times; that care in the neurorehabilitation facility raises those odds by 10.45 times and for those in the 'after' group, i.e. receiving the new service, by 4.31 times. All these odds are 'adjusted' odds ratios, i.e. they are adjusted for other main effects in the model, so for example the raised odds of 4.31 times for the new service takes into account the raised odds caused by the neurorehabilitation service. This statistical model provides the first tentative evidence to suggest that the new pattern of service delivery is having an effect on the packages of care constructed, supporting the patterns of care shown in the case histories.

What though about quality of life issues such as social isolation? The case histories imply potential for improvement in these areas. Examining the impact of the new service by looking at social isolation (i.e. any positive score on the NHP subscale), a logistic regression equation shows that the need for psychological intervention, as expressed by a score of five or above on the GHQ 28, raises the odds of being socially isolated by 42.6 times! However, other factors are working to reduce these odds. Time to follow-up does so, by 1.07 times per month, suggesting that while other factors are held constant, as time passes (certainly in the short term) social isolation will decrease. The presence of the community OT also reduces the odds of being socially isolated by 3.7 times. Thus once again the presence of the community OTs do seem to be having an effect on outcome, in this case levels of social isolation, and this lends further empirical support to the type of networking activity evident in the case histories above.

Further evidence to support the positive impact of the project can be derived from tentative models predicting carer's emotional reactions. The NHP emotional reaction subscale includes items such as 'Things are getting me down' and 'I'm feeling on edge'. A logistic regression model found that the carer's emotional wellbeing is worsened by an above-average carer-perceived sequelae score, as well as when an RTA is the cause of the injury. Presence of the community OT reduced the likelihood of having a positive (worse) score by 2.27 times. In this instance though, the number of carers reduced the power of the model to show a significant difference, hence the 'tentative' label.

Taking the reduction in social isolation for the client, the tentative evidence to suggest improvement in quality of life dimensions for the carer, together with the increased package of care associated with the presence of the community OT and the qualitative case histories which set these activities in real-life context, there is support for the contention that the new model of care improves coordination of service delivery and some aspects of the quality of life of the head-injured family.

The effect of the lack of these apparently simple service improvements is well illustrated by the case of James, a 35-year-old, injured in a road traffic accident and discharged in April 1989 after 30 days stay. When he was visited a year following discharge, James and his wife were deep in debt. Because of dizziness he was unable to walk further than his garden and they could see no hope for the future. James's wife said, 'What goes on after . . .? It's just like getting tortured. Everything was so good in hospital.' They had received no visit to their home since James's discharge.

SERVICE IMPLICATIONS

With one in three OTs in the UK now working in the community, there is considerable scope for using our model as a practical means of community reintegration for those discharged after a head injury. To be effective

OTs must have management support, dedicated time for this work and be fully trained in TBI. Such a model of service has costs and a case has to be made for the use of resources to run it.

In some countries OTs are scarce and replication of this initiative may be difficult given the range of skills displayed by these community OTs. However, even though attention will have to be paid to obtaining comprehensive assessments, the 'safety net' and networking roles could be undertaken by most community professionals, given the resources and knowledge of local services.

The average cost of this service in terms of community OT time is about £300 ($450) per case. Development and training time likely to be incurred by any agency wishing to replicate this initiative will have to be budgeted for, and this cost does not diminish, given staff turnover and the need to keep abreast of developments in treatment. Indirect costs, such as capital expenditure, management costs and so on, will vary between areas and agencies.

The range of resources that can be utilized to help is also likely to vary between districts, some of which have better developed services than others. The greater the range of local resources the greater the chance of providing effective community reintegration without referral out of the district. It is probably fair to say that the results of the current project have arisen mostly because of the assessment, referral, networking and 'case management' style work rather, than a major extension of the time given to therapy, for example, in developing memory training or similar modalities of treatment. In many respects, the project gave the OTs 'space' to be able to use their broad range of skills, with additional emphasis given to networking and coordinating packages of care. The value of providing this opportunity is, we feel, amply demonstrated by the case histories and research findings.

Thus, we believe that our model, with its emphasis on full assessment, and the use of existing services in health, social care and education, is worthy of consideration in many localities and cultures. Its flexibility and scientific base allow both for quantification and evaluation and also, most probably, for a most effective and cost-effective use of scarce resources.

REFERENCES

1. Murphy LD, McMillan TM, Greenwood RJ et al. Services for severely head-injured patients in North London and environs. Brain Injury 1990; 4: 95–100.
2. Cockburn JM, Gatherer A. Facilities for rehabilitation of adults after head injury. Clinical Rehabilitation 1988; 2: 315–318.
3. Edwards FC, Warren MD. Health Services for Adults with Physical Disabilities. London: Royal College of Physicians of London, 1990.
4. Chamberlain MA (Chairman). The Ideal Management of Head Injury. Leeds: West Yorkshire Working Party, 1988.

5. The Disabled Persons (Services, Consultation and Representation) Act. London: HMSO, 1986.
6. Department of Health and Social Security. *Caring for People*. London: HMSO, 1989.
7. Wade DT. Policies on the management of patients with head injury: the experience of Oxford Region. *Clinical Rehabilitation* 1991; **5**: 141–155.
8. Kreutzer JS, Zasler ND, Camplair PS *et al*. A practical guide to family intervention following adult traumatic brain injury. In: Kreutzer JS, Wehman P, eds. *Community Integration Following Traumatic Brain Injury*. Sevenoaks: Edward Arnold, 1990: pp 249–273.
9. Teasdale G, Jennett B. Assessment of coma and impaired consciousness. A practical scale. *Lancet* 1974; **ii**: 81–83.
10. Jennett B, Bond M. Assessment of outcome after severe brain damage. A practical scale. *Lancet* 1975; **i**: 480–484.
11. World Health Organization. *The International Classification of Impairments Disabilities and Handicaps*. Geneva: World Health Organization, 1980.
12. Mahoney FI, Barthel DW. Functional evaluation: the Barthel Index. *Maryland State Medical Journal* 1965; **14**: 61–65.
13. Cooper B, Shah S, Vanclay F. Improving the sensitivity of the BARTHEL Index for stroke rehabilitation. *Journal of Clinical Epidemiology* 1989; **42**: 703–709.
14. Hunt SM, McEwan J, McKenna SP. Measuring health status: a new tool for clinicians and epidemiologists. *Journal of the Royal College of General Practitioners* 1985; **35**: 185–188.
15. Hunt SM, McEwen J, McKenna SP. *Measuring Health Status*. London: Croom Helm, 1986.
16. Dick JPR, Guiloff RJ, Stewart A *et al*. Mini-mental state examination in neurological patients. *Journal of Neurology, Neurosurgery, and Psychiatry* 1984; **47**: 496–499.
17. Whiting SE, Lincoln NB, Bhavnani G *et al*. *The Rivermead Perceptual Assessment Battery*. Windsor: NFER-Nelson, 1980.
18. Intagliata J. Improving the quality of community care for the chronically mentally disabled: the role of case management. *Schizophrenia Bulletin* 1982; **8**: 655–674.
19. Eames P, Wood RL. The structure and content of a head injury rehabilitation service. In: Wood RL, Eames P, eds. *Models of Brain Injury Rehabilitation*. London: Chapman & Hall, 1988.
20. Goldberg DP, Hillier VF. A scaled version of the General Health Questionnaire. *Psychological Medicine* 1979; **9**: 139–145.
21. Glantz SA, Slinker BK. *Primer of Applied Regression and Analysis of Variance*. New York: McGraw-Hill, 1990.
22. Collet D. *Modelling Binary Data*. London: Chapman & Hall, 1991.

A home-based service:

a community rehabilitation programme

7

Miroslav Palát and Miroslav Palát Jr

INTRODUCTION

The number of persons suffering from disabling or potentially disabling conditions is steadily increasing. In the main they are either the victims of acute events, such as road traffic accidents and sport injuries, or patients in the terminal stage of a chronic disabling and/or mutilating disease. Both present a considerable challenge to contemporary rehabilitation medicine.

The aim of rehabilitation medicine is to restore or maintain those functions of the organism that have been compromised by an underlying pathology. Rehabilitation programmes use distinct means and methods of rehabilitation, which aim at the improvement of individual functions of the organism, as well as the wellbeing of the entire person – a more complex task. Comprehensive rehabilitation programmes consider also the psychological and social impact of an impairment, which ultimately affect the quality of life. Patients with either temporary or permanent disabilities need rehabilitation care, but many are insufficiently mobile to reach the rehabilitation unit.

Within a structured, comprehensive rehabilitation approach there may be a number of components that do not necessarily require the equipment of a hospital rehabilitation department. Our thrust towards a home-based rehabilitation programme arose for two reasons. More flexibility in rehabilitation care is desirable; we also have to address the challenge of an ever increasing number of patients suitable for such treatment. There were also various practicalities and financial aspects.

The home-based rehabilitation programme has saved the immobile patient from the difficulties of being transported to and from the rehabilitation department of the local hospital. It was, instead, the physio-therapist who took on the travelling and administered the rehabilitation treatment at the patient's home.

The indications for domiciliary treatment included neurological disorders resulting from head and/or spine injuries, multiple trauma, lower limb fractures, stroke and a variety of other neurological disorders. The indications for such a programme related to the underlying disease and the functional condition found on examination.

SETTING

The home-based rehabilitation programme scheme took place in Bratislava, then in Czechoslovakia, now the capital of the Slovak Republic. This is a city with a population of 500 000. The project has been put into practice within the structures of the municipal health authority. It was a model study, which started in 1980 and went on for 5 years.

A basic ambulance van provided the means of transport used and was organized by the hospital ambulance service. The crew included the driver and one physiotherapist trained in the appropriate methods and techniques.

The physiotherapists were members of the hospital rehabilitation department staff and they were allocated to this particular task, usually for a period of 3 months. The increasing number of programmes performed during home visits corresponds with more city districts being included in the scheme year after year.

HOW IT WORKED

The physician at the hospital rehabilitation clinic decided on the scope, extent and frequency of the rehabilitation programme. This decision was based on a complete clinical examination, X-ray and biochemical and functional assessments.

Patients who had been found suitable for the first phase of the rehabil-itation programme were included in the scheme. After this a thorough check-up at the hospital was performed. It included all aspects mentioned above, with the aim of determining the clinical condition and its potential for improvement. According to the results the home-based programme was adjusted and continued.

The patient was seen by the physiotherapist two to three times a week, one physiotherapist looking after four to eight patients. In the course of the project, the city area was divided into five districts (with 50 000–70 000 inhabitants each); each of these was looked after by one team derived from the respective rehabilitation departments of district hospitals.

Progress was evaluated by the physiotherapist at the end of each session two to three times per week. The hospital rehabilitation physician saw the patient and checked the progress once a month. The physician also decided when the home-based programme was to be terminated and the patient would be able to complete his/her rehabilitation treatment on an out-patient basis.

BENEFITS

Within our 5-year experience with this model study 30 094 rehabilitation programmes have been conducted. On the patients' side notable benefits were recorded. Patients enjoyed their treatment in a homely environment. A disabled person is usually closely attached to the environment he/she is used to.

There was a great potential for gaining the family's assistance in the process. The involvement of family members in the rehabilitation process was encouraged by educating individuals to carry out some exercises with their relatives themselves. This has strongly increased the likelihood of the relatives participating actively in the rehabilitation treatment. Thus, some procedures were carried out with increased frequency even in the physiotherapist's absence. With the relatives involved, there was an overall improvement of compliance. This resulted in an apparent gradual improvement in the patients' condition.

For the municipal health authority there were also strong considerations, particularly on the side of the ambulance service. If an immobile patient needed to be transported to and from the rehabilitation treatment, this would involve a mean distance of roughly 25 km per patient, whereas patients visited by the physiotherapists would only rarely require transport to the hospital, so that the mean distance came down to as low as 6–8 km per patient per treatment. There was a considerable saving of money and time by the use of a properly designed and conducted home-based rehabilitation programme.

SHORTCOMINGS

A home-based programme cannot entirely replace a comprehensive programme, which has to be carried out in specialized institutes with all due facilities. Some compromises also have to be made to enable the best possible use of the physiotherapists' time. Nevertheless, this has been optimized by a thorough preparation of the itinerary. Unexpected problems also occurred when insufficient compliance on the relatives' side was encountered. This proved to be a rare but considerable setback in the treatment's progress.

CONCLUSIONS

The scheme has, so far, only been proved to be suitable for densely populated, urban communities with 60 000 inhabitants or more.

It could also prove useful in areas or boroughs with no regional rehabilitation medicine department or one insufficiently equipped. Naturally, a well-equipped rehabilitation department provides means that far exceed the home-based programmes.

It is doubtful if such a scheme is practicable in rural areas, where the benefits would not compensate for the large amount of time spent by the qualified physiotherapist in travelling or for the running costs of the vehicle.

Overall, the home-based rehabilitation programme has proved to be a valuable alternative to hospital rehabilitation care, if it is performed under the right conditions and within the context of a comprehensive rehabilitation approach.

A clinically and neurophysiologically led postacute rehabilitation programme

8

Anne-Lise Christensen and
Thomas Teasdale

INTRODUCTION

The Centre for Rehabilitation of Brain Injury was established by the first author (ALC) in 1985, initially with funding from the Danish Egmont Foundation, to provide a rehabilitation service to postacute brain-injured adults. At that time, no such facility existed in Denmark. The history of the Centre can, however, be traced further back to the late 1960s, when ALC, then a clinical psychologist in a neurosurgical department, encountered the works of A. R. Luria, in particular, his *Higher Cortical Functions in Man* [1]. Three visits to Luria's clinic in Moscow culminated in the first systematic presentation of Luria's neuropsychological investigation techniques [2]. By the late 1980s rehabilitation centres were beginning to emerge in the United States, and ALC visited several of these, particularly those of Ben-Yishay in New York and Prigatano, then in Oklahoma. At the time that the establishment of the Copenhagen centre was being negotiated, ALC was working in a hospital psychiatry department, but it was decided that a rehabilitation centre such as the one envisaged would best be located outside a medical environment, so the collaboration and hospitality of Copenhagen University's Psychological Laboratory was sought and was kindly forthcoming. The university setting has led to our referring to the people entering our programme as *lever*, which can be translated as 'students', but in the present context we shall refer to them as 'clients'.

Although the organization and structure of the Centre's rehabilitation programme has changed in numerous important ways in the subsequent 7 years, some basic elements remain largely unchanged, as have its objectives. The Centre aims to rehabilitate, in the neuropsychological, physical and social senses of this term, clients who have suffered a brain injury. In order to be admitted to the programme, they must (usually) meet a number of inclusion and exclusion criteria. The injury must have an identified aetiology and have had an acute onset. The most common groups fulfilling these criteria are those having suffered head injury or stroke. Degenerative disorders such as Alzheimer's disease are generally an excluded diagnostic category, since their problems are of a radically different nature and prognosis. Children under the age of 16 are also excluded, mainly because of developmental changes surrounding puberty. The Centre does not impose any upper age limit, but in practice, as will be explained below, local authority social service departments are rarely willing to fund anyone over the age of 55. Potential clients must have attained a reasonable level of school education, mental retardation being an exclusion criterion. They must be motivated for treatment and they should preferably have a supporting family or social environment. There should be a potential for improvement of intellectual, emotional and psychosocial functioning, optimally with a view to subsequent re-employment or further education. In part owing to these latter requirements, alcoholism, drug abuse or severe mental illness are also exclusion criteria.

Referrals to the Centre can be made by a general practitioner, a hospital department or a public authority. Referrals must be accompanied by medical information regarding the origin and course of the injury, and, on the basis of the information, the potential client will be called in for a preliminary examination. All referrals to the Centre are evaluated by a review committee, including senior physicians which also advises on problematic cases. The committee members comprise a rheumatologist, a neurologist, a neurosurgeon, a psychiatrist, two of the Centre's psychologists (including ALC) and a referrals administrator.

Irrespective of who makes the initial referral, the cost of the programme has most often been met by the social services department of the local authority region (*kommune*) in which the client resides. In a few cases insurance companies have met the expense. The programme, including the extensive follow-up, currently costs 215 000 Danish kroner (approximately £20 000). At present negotiations are proceeding with the national Ministry of Health to secure an arrangement whereby the Centre will be guaranteed a viable number of funded places annually.

Most clients enter the programme at one year or more post injury. In some cases, especially for those having suffered an injury in infancy or childhood, the interval can be much longer. A typical course will be an acute admission into an orthopaedic or neurosurgical department, followed by a longer period of physical rehabilitation in a rheumatological hospital. In the early years very few of our clients came directly from rheumatology, although more recently this has become commoner. Many have made attempts to return to their working lives and have experienced greater or lesser degrees of failure in this. None of our clients are engaged in employment or an educational programme at the time they begin the programme, although some have the opportunity to return to their former activity conditional upon a successful rehabilitation.

Prior to entering the programme, clients are invited to a preliminary assessment in which their suitability for acceptance into the programme is evaluated. A core element in this assessment is the Luria Neuropsychological Investigation [1], in which clients' deficits are identified, and no less importantly their remaining intact functions, since these form a cornerstone of the rehabilitation process. On the basis of the assessment, together with previously gathered anamnestic and epicrisis medical information, a detailed report is sent to the appropriate local authority caseworker.

The staffing of the Centre reflects the conscious attempt to create an educational rather than a medical environment. There are currently nine clinical- and neuro-psychologists, including the director (ALC), two physiotherapists, two speech therapists (one specializing in aphasias and the other in dysarthrias) and a special education teacher. In addition, the staff include three secretaries, a book-keeper and a practical administrator. In addition to the medical specialists serving on the review committee, a consultant neurologist examines all of the clients when they start the programme and when they finish it. The Centre has, furthermore, very wide contacts within the neurological fields of medicine in Copenhagen and across Denmark, and *ad hoc* consultations regarding particular cases are not uncommon. The emphasis on psychological rather than medical rehabilitation reflects the widely established finding that the psychological problems following a brain injury are the most chronic and the most intractable [3–5].

THE REHABILITATION PROGRAMME

The rehabilitation programme itself has two phases, a 4–5 month intensive programme phase, succeeded by an extended follow-up period of at least 6 months. Clients are admitted to the programme simultaneously in groups of about 10–15. The programmes run approximately simultaneously with the university's two annual terms, i.e. one in spring–summer and one in autumn–winter. The centre is non-resident and clients come for four days per week, Tuesday through Friday, for 6 hours per day (09:00–15:00).

In the first few days of the programme, the clients are examined using a semi-structured psychosocial interview, a wide range of psychological tests (e.g. the Wechsler Adult Intelligence Scale, Ravens Progressive Matrices, subtests of the Wechsler Memory Scale, the Rorschach ink-blot test), and standardized psychological and psychosocial questionnaires (the Katz Social Adjustment Scale, Syndrome Check List and an Activities of Daily Living scale). Some of the latter are also completed by a near relative or close acquaintance.

Much of this testing is conducted by the psychologist, who is given primary responsibility for following the client through the programme and thereafter. Allocation of particular psychologists to particular clients is made prior to the start of the programme on the basis of anticipated compatibilities etc.. The allocation is not, however, necessarily adhered to rigidly thereafter and some readjustments may take place during the course of the programme.

Each day of the programme begins with a morning meeting of 30 minutes duration, attended by all of the clients and three of the staff. The meeting has a rather fixed agenda, which includes any alterations in the programme for the day, a set of simple physical exercises and a review of major items from the television news of the previous evening. The meeting concludes with a 'morning song' chosen from a widely used book of folk songs. In the first few weeks the staff members conduct this meeting, but thereafter responsibilities are delegated to the clients themselves. Thus one client will be responsible for chairing the meeting, one for leading the physical exercises, one for presenting the news items and one for minuting the meeting. Immediate feedback is given to these clients from both the staff and other clients regarding their performance.

On a typical day the morning meeting will be followed by a session of individual cognitive training. This activity can take a wide variety of forms, depending on the particular client. These can include the use of computerized training programmes stimulating concentration and attention, sustained tempo, memory, reasoning ability, problem solving, planning and structuring. It is important to emphasize, however, that close observation and interaction are maintained during training, in order that qualitative aspects of the client's performance, including motivation and affective state, can be noted and guided and that the client can obtain a personal feedback regarding his/her performance. Cognitive training can also be concerned with practical details of the client's everyday life. All clients are, for instance, issued with an appointments diary when they begin the programme and a ring-binder in which to sort and file the various documents and notes that they receive. Cognitive training can encompass the effective use of these resources. Where appropriate, clients may be taught or retaught the rudiments of word processing, at which most of the staff have some proficiency. For aphasic clients much of the cognitive training is concentrated upon restoring their language skills.

Another important element of the programme is group psychotherapy, and sessions take place twice weekly. The clients are divided into a younger and an older group. The psychotherapy sessions for both groups are led by two psychologists, who do not have individual responsibility for the clients in the group. In these sessions the clients discuss and share with each other the experiences and feelings that have surrounded their injury, the ways in which it has affected their lives and how they are learning to overcome or accommodate to the difficulties which it has brought in its wake. Some individual sessions of the client with his or her psychologist can also be used to deal with personal problems in particular crises which have arisen or are threatening.

Physical training takes place several times a week and serves more than one function. In part it helps to restore the often much neglected physical condition of the clients, who in many cases have been physically inactive since their injury. But, since the training is planned to follow precisely established and structured routines, it supplements the cognitive training and since it is a group activity, it further promotes social interaction between the clients. The university buildings do not have good facilities for physical training, and the fitness club of a nearby large hotel is therefore used (where the clients mingle freely with hotel guests), although some activities, including volleyball and a dance session (using the highly structured 'Lancers' dance), do take place on our premises.

Some of the physical training overlaps areas that might elsewhere be the province of ergotherapy. Thus it can involve relearning the skill of bicycling or learning to use a tricycle. Some clients participate in a weekly cooking class, especially the younger ones, who may be establishing independent living, and home visits are often arranged early in the course of the programme, particularly for those clients who live alone, in order to view and, where necessary, to help improve their living conditions. Both the physiotherapists and other staff members may become involved in training in the use of bus and train services for those clients who initially must be brought to and from the Centre by private transport.

The week ends with a lecture, which all the clients attend. The initial lectures are given by staff members or consultants and cover topics of immediate relevance to the clients, such as the functional organization of the brain and the nature and consequences of their various forms of brain injury. Thereafter they are given by invited experts and usually include nutrition, exercise, sexuality, handicap sports, journalism and the media. At one invited lecture former clients are invited to talk about their experiences of the programme and subsequent to it.

In addition to these activities, a very important element of the programme is contact with family members. This contact is established at a welcoming reception held at the beginning of the programme to which relatives are invited. They are invited to attend meetings, arranged by ALC and one other staff member, held in the late afternoon once a fortnight through the course of the programme. The clients themselves do not attend these meetings and the focus of attention is on the relatives' own experiences of and reactions to their family member's brain injury and its aftermath. The meetings are held in a relaxed and informal atmosphere with no agenda, and two separate groups are usually formed, one comprising spouses or partners to the older clients and the other comprising parents of the younger ones. The objectives of these meetings are to promote an understanding and acceptance of the injury that has befallen the family.

Throughout the course of the programme weekly full staff meetings are held, at which the cases of individual clients in turn are reviewed at length, progress is monitored and solutions for rectifying any problems that have arisen are discussed and agreed upon.

During the early stages of the programme, emphasis is placed upon dealing with strengthening the client's cognitive, emotional and social resources. Thereafter, and increasingly towards the end of the 4–5 month period, stress is placed on the client's life after completion of the programme. Arrangements may be made early for independent living facilities (possibly sheltered accommodation or rooms in a hall of residence), particularly for the younger clients for whom brain injury has necessitated a return to the parental home. New and/or former spare-time hobbies and pastimes are promoted.

Of special importance to many clients is their prospects for employment or further education. This issue needs to be approached with sensitivity, since almost all of the clients were in employment or an educational programme at the time of their injury, and most have aspirations to return to it in some form. Where the practical opportunity is present, and where the client's abilities are deemed sufficient, an attempt is made to achieve a return to the former employment. Occasionally, the former place of employment is able to provide a niche where less demand is placed on the client, perhaps with the prospect of increasing the level of involvement with the passage of time. Unfortunately, these options are not always open, and much effort is therefore concentrated upon finding feasible alternatives. The task is hampered by the high level of unemployment in Denmark, but it is often possible to find some form of meaningful and rewarding occupation for the client, either in state-sponsored workshops, etc. or in employment in regular workplaces, with a wage subsidized by the state as an incentive to the employer.

The completion of the programme is marked by intensive assessment, largely involving the same battery of procedures, i.e. interviews and tests, described above for the beginning of the programme. In order to increase objectivity, some of the testing, both before and after the programme, is conducted by a psychologist not employed at the Centre.

On the basis of the assessment results and the course of the programme in general, a comprehensive report is sent to the client's local authority, to his/her general practitioner and to the client him/herself.

FOLLOW-UP

As stated above, contact with the clients does not terminate at the end of the day programme. In collaboration with social department caseworkers, the negotiations and procedures concerning employment, education or accommodation that have already been initiated are followed through, particularly by the psychologist with primary responsibility for the client. Meetings for the whole group are arranged on a monthly basis for 6 months following the completion of the programme. At these meetings, which are usually very well attended and which are guided by two of the Centre's staff, the clients have an opportunity to exchange information about what has been happening to them. Almost all of the clients also return at varying intervals for meetings lasting about an hour with the staff members with whom they were most involved. In some cases, notably the aphasics, these are arranged on a regular basis, perhaps weekly, as a direct continuation of the rehabilitation process.

Some forms of social activity are also offered to former clients. A course of theoretical and practical instruction in sailing is given weekly, and a chess and backgammon club flourishes. A film club and a book club (particularly for those with aphasia) are currently being planned.

At 1 year and at 3 years after the completion of the programme, all clients are invited to return to the Centre for a day of interviewing and testing, a day in which time is also scheduled for more informal social interaction.

It is important to emphasize that the Centre has an open-door policy towards former clients and many do indeed contact the Centre up to several years later in order to obtain help in some particular situation, such as, perhaps, entering a new educational programme or because of marital conflict.

The extensive assessment of the clients at the beginning of the programme is used for the clinical purpose of deciding upon a specific rehabilitation strategy. However, it is also used, in combination with that undertaken at the end of the programme and those at 1 and 3 years after it, for the research purpose of measuring outcome. Neuropsychological test results typically show some gains, although often with a residual deficiency relative to population norms. Our main interest, as much in research as clinically, has however concentrated upon psychosocial outcome, i.e. valid measures of the important aspects of the daily life of the client. Three of our major concerns under this heading have been independent living arrangements, employment or education, and hobbies and pastimes.

RESULTS

As stated above, the Centre opened in 1985 and by 1988 a total of 67 clients had completed the programme. We shall here present results, up to the 3-year follow-up, of outcome for these clients. These data derive from our own interviews, supplemented by reference to the medical records and to relatives and social workers. The results are reported more fully elsewhere [6].

Of the 67 clients, 61% were male. Over 50% had suffered head injury and 30% had suffered stroke. The average age at injury was 24 years and on average a further 2 years elapsed before they entered the programme.

The home circumstances of the clients were at all times highly diverse. We have, however, grouped them into three major categories. The first of these is the condition of living with a spouse (or cohabitant), the second is living alone and independently and the third is living in a 'dependent' situation, such as continuing (or returning) to live with parents or other close relatives, living in sheltered accommodation, etc. Given the fact that the very large majority of our clients were over the age of 18 by the time of completion of the programme, this scale may be regarded as ordinal.

Figure 8.1 shows the distribution of these categories at five time points.

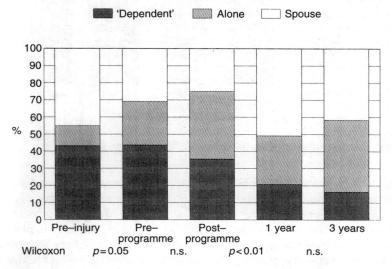

Figure 8.1 Domestic situation from pre-injury to 3 years post-programme.

It can be seen that there is a significant change in the pattern following injury. The proportion living in marital or other partner relationships declined, reflecting the fact that such relationships are often placed under heavy strain by the brain injury of one of the partners. The fact that the proportion in 'dependent' situations remained the same is probably because an otherwise natural tendency for the youngest of our clients to leave the parental home had been arrested by the occurrence of the injury. There is no significant change during the 4–5 months of the programme itself but by the 1-year follow-up the pattern had significantly altered in the direction of many fewer living in dependent situations and many more living in partner relationships. It is noteworthy that there was no significant change between the 1-year and 3-year follow-up, i.e. although no further improvements were found neither was there any evidence of a decline back towards the preprogramme conditions.

Figure 8.2 shows the situation regarding occupation.

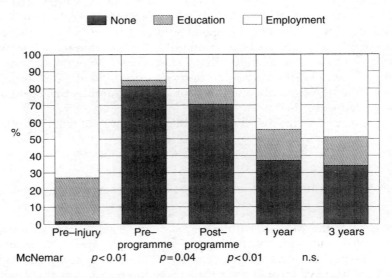

Figure 8.2 Occupation from pre-injury to 3 years post-programme.

Here too we have grouped a variety of different circumstances into three major categories, namely in some form of employment (part or full-time, competitive wage earning or subsidized), in an educational programme or neither of these. As can be seen, virtually all clients were in employment or education at the time of the injury. At the start of the programme, virtually none were. The small percentage, who technically were 'employed' were receiving sickness benefit and had no assurance of returning to their original jobs unless rehabilitation was successful. Immediately after leaving the programme and continuing up to 1 year after, there was a significant decline in the numbers of 'inactive' clients. At the 1-year follow-up over 60% were employed or engaged in an educational programme. As with the domestic situation, there were no further changes, either for better or worse, between the 1-year and 3-year follow-ups.

Figure 8.3 shows the distribution of reported hobbies and leisure activities.

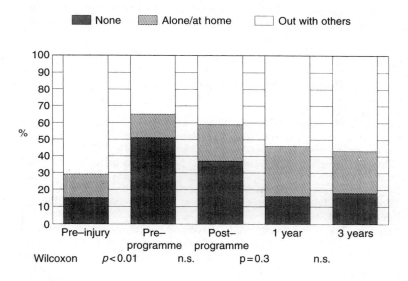

Figure 8.3 Leisure activities from pre-injury to 3 years post-programme.

In view of the well-known tendency of brain-injured people towards withdrawal and social isolation, we have been especially interested in the degree of social activity involved in leisure activities. Again, therefore, we have formed a simple trichotomy comprising those whose leisure activities take them out of their own home and into the company of others, those whose activities take place either alone and/or at home and those for whom no hobbies or leisure activities are reported. This variable can also be treated as an ordinal scale, and as such a significant decline is seen between pre-injury and preprogramme. As can be seen a picture similar to that for the other two variables emerges. There is a significant decline in leisure activities following injury. The pattern does not change during the course of the programme, but leisure activities, particularly those which are social and outside of the home, increase significantly up to follow-up at 1 year. Between 1 year and 3 years the pattern of leisure activities is also stable.

These three variables show a common pattern: declining function following injury, a recovery after entering the programme up to 1 year after its completion and a stable status thereafter. Taken together with the fact that the gains appear to be unrelated to time since injury, the very fact of the stability supports two encouraging conclusions. The first is that it is the programme itself that has produced the changes, since a pattern of spontaneous recovery would not have been confined to the period between, on average 2 years post-injury and 3.5 years post-injury. The second is that the gains produced by the programme do not, as is often feared in rehabilitation work, fade with time, but remain stable.

REFERENCES

1. Luria AR. *Higher Cortical Functions in Man*. New York: Basic Books, 1980.
2. Christensen A-L. *Luria's Neuropsychological Investigation*. Copenhagen: Munksgaard, 1975.
3. McKinlay WW, Brooks DN, Bond MR *et al*. The short-term outcome of severe blunt head injury as reported by relatives of injured persons. *Journal of Neurology, Neurosurgery, and Neuropsychiatry* 1981; **44**: 527.
4. Oddy M, Coughlan T, Tyerman A *et al*. Social adjustment after closed-head injury: A further follow-up seven years after injury. *Journal of Neurology, Neurosurgery, and Neuropsychiatry*, 1985; **48**: 564–568.
5. Thomsen IV. Late psychosocial outcome in severe blunt head injury. *Brain Injury* 1987; **1**: 131–143.
6. Teasdale TW, Christensen A-L. Psychosocial outcome in Denmark. In: Christensen A-L, Uzzell B, eds. *Brain Injury and Neuropsychological Rehabilitation: International Perspectives*.). Hillsdale, NJ: Lawrence Erlbaum Associates, 1993: pp 235–244.

PART TWO

Recent initiatives in traumatic brain injury rehabilitation

Principles and practice of treatment

9

Vera C. Neumann

INTRODUCTION

The scale of the problem presented by traumatic brain injury (TBI) has been discussed in the first section of this book, often using melodramatic terms such as 'the silent epidemic'. These terms are appropriate, for TBI represents a huge health problem, causing more deaths in men aged 18–30 in Western Europe than any other illness or injury.

Whereas the first part of this book describes ways of approaching the management of TBI in population terms, this section deals with the management of the problems faced by individuals who have suffered head injuries and by their families and friends.

Two further points should be made. This section covers management of non-penetrating head injuries, the type most commonly encountered by its European authors. The problems specifically associated with penetrating head wounds are not covered. Experience of dealing with these is greater in the United States, and the interested reader should therefore refer to American texts on this subject. Secondly, emphasis is placed on the treatment of severe head injuries rather than the numerically much more frequent mild or moderate injuries.

THE PATTERNS OF PATHOLOGY

Since TBI is usually the consequence of an accident or assault, and chance determines where the head is struck, one might expect the pattern of pathology to show great variety. If this were so, one would also expect to see a very variable spectrum of impairments and it would therefore be difficult to generalize about treatment. In fact, certain pathological features are commonly seen irrespective of the site of the impact. These are described in the following paragraphs and, as indicated below, their nature and distribution are in part influenced by the laws of physics.

EFFECTS OF IMPACT: RAPID ACCELERATION OR DECELERATION

The brain is a soft structure, enclosed within the rigid skull and partly tethered to it. Energy transferred to the skull during impact has to be dissipated within the head. This results in twisting and oscillating movements of the brain, with two main effects on the brain tissue itself. Firstly, rotational and other movements within the brain shear structures, particularly where movement is maximal. Areas linking more mobile structures with tethered parts, such as the proximal brain stem and corpus callosum, can be expected to bear the brunt of these shear forces. Within the brain tissue, the structures most likely to be torn are long, thin structures such as long neuronal axons or exposed, partially tethered blood vessels.

Secondly, impact occurs between the brain and the skull. The internal surface of the skull, particularly underneath the frontal lobes and temporal poles, is rough, with numerous bony spikes and ridges. These can lacerate the soft brain as it rubs against them, causing contusions. Other areas, such as the smoother cranial vaults, would be less likely to cause this sort of damage. This theoretical pattern of damage was first demonstrated by Holbourn using gelatine models [1]. Post-mortem studies on subjects who have died from their injuries [1] and, more recently, neuroimaging techniques such as CT or MRI scans have confirmed this pattern.

EFFECTS OF COMPRESSION

Following a severe closed head injury, blood from blood vessels damaged by direct injury, shear or oedema from damaged tissues must either be removed or controlled (perhaps by neurosurgical intervention) or must lead to further damage by compression. Again, the laws of physics determine where this causes the most harm. When the brain is forced against the cranial vaults, the surface area is large and the pressure in any one area is therefore relatively small. When instead the brain is forced down against the sharp, rigid edge of the tentorium, the area of contact is small; pressures generated are therefore high and local damage is likely to occur. The third cranial nerve is particularly vulnerable here; hence the usefulness of monitoring its function by checking pupillary constriction in the unconscious patient who has had recent trauma.

EFFECTS OF ISCHAEMIA AND HYPOTENSION

One consequence of raised intracranial pressure is impaired tissue perfusion; if pressure in brain tissue exceeds that in the capillaries this is inevitable. However, a more important cause of ischaemic damage is impaired perfusion due to hypovolaemic shock. Simply because many who sustain traumatic brain injuries also sustain injuries elsewhere, shock is common. Furthermore, injuries to the chest or airways obstruction may mean that blood reaching the brain is also poorly oxygenated, aggravating the effects of ischaemia still further.

Once again this produces a typical pattern of damage, this time determined by the vascular supply of the brain as well as its physical properties. Areas supplied by vessels that lie adjacent to rigid structures and are thus compressed if intracranial pressure rises, and watershed areas between adjacent vascular supplies, are the most vulnerable. The posterior parietal lobes may, for example, suffer ischaemic damage in this way. This secondary damage due to ischaemia and hypoxia is numerically important. This combination has been shown to increase mortality threefold [2], and outcome in survivors (in terms of return to work or education) is also correspondingly worse [3].

EXTENSION OF NEUROLOGICAL DAMAGE

One commonly seen sequela is diffuse atrophy; ventricular enlargement indicative of such atrophy has been detected by neuroimaging in as many as 70% of head-injured patients [4]. Atrophy tends to be bilateral, even if the initial injury has been associated with a unilateral problem such as a haematoma. Although atrophy associated with increased ventricular size is frequently noted in scans 2–3 months after the initial injury, this does not indicate high-pressure post-traumatic hydrocephalus, and shunting is seldom required (less than 6% in Gudeman's series) [5]. Instead, secondary degeneration of neurones that have lost their synaptic connections probably accounts for much of this atrophy.

It follows from the above that, although the site of impact and direct damage will vary greatly, certain pathological features and therefore certain signs and symptoms (impairments) are demonstrable in many cases of TBI.

Before proceeding to discuss these impairments and the consequent disabilities and handicaps, it is worth noting that the abnormalities detectable by imaging techniques such as CT or MRI scans are not necessarily those responsible for the functional impairments. Diffuse axonal injury, for example, may be associated with severe disability but initially normal CT scans [6]. On the other hand, contusions, which are readily visible as haemorrhagic areas on CT scans, may have few neurological consequences. Some 3–4% of the general population have evidence of cerebral contusions at autopsy, irrespective of the cause of death [7]. In fact, the only scan feature that seems to correlate with psychological impairment is ventricular volume at 2–3 months [8]. Nevertheless, the argument that common patterns of pathology and common patterns of impairment can be identified irrespective of the site of impact still holds true.

For this reason it is possible to predict certain disabilities (disturbances of function) characteristic of TBI (Table 9.1). This and the following chapters take advantage of this common ground and describe ways of minimizing these disabilities and consequent handicaps.

Table 9.1 Problems characteristic of severe traumatic brain injury

Physical problems

- Coma
- Fits
- Disorders of movement
- Disorders of sensation
- Disorders of speech and/or swallowing
- Incontinence

Cognitive problems

- Attention/slow information processing
- Memory problems
- Language/communication problems
- Visual and other perceptual problems
- Executive function problems

Emotional problems

- Anxiety and/or depression
- Apathy
- Disinhibition (sexual/social)
- Modulation of emotion (blunting and/or lability)
- Egocentricity/lack of empathy

MINIMIZING DISABILITY AND HANDICAP

Management will be considered under the following headings.

- The early phase, where the focus is on minimizing disabilities;
- the transitional phase, where the focus is on matching skills (particularly cognitive and behavioural) to the anticipated needs at home;
- the community phase, during which the focus is on achieving new goals, and adjustment.

GENERAL REMARKS

Rehabilitation is not a cure. It is a means of enabling a person to circumvent persistent impairments in order to minimize disability and handicap. By the time the rehabilitation team first encounters a patient with TBI, the extent of neurological impairment will probably already have been determined. There is considerable scope for influencing the extent of such impairments, and efforts should be made to do so. Changes in the organization and quality of trauma services may do much to minimize particularly secondary damage due to hypoxia and hypotension [2,9]. New drugs, such as those that limit damage produced by glutamate released from injured neural tissue, the so-called NMDA antagonists, and new techniques such as neurotransplantation also offer some hope for minimizing impairments in the very early stages. However, in this book we are concerned with the rehabilitation process once the medical condition has stabilized.

This chapter describes management particularly of physical problems, while the other authors in this section describe their personal approaches to the management of cognitive and behavioural problems. Although the rehabilitation process has been divided in this way, for it to be successful the process must be multidisciplinary. Assessments should be carried out by a team whose professional skills encompass occupational therapy, physiotherapy, speech therapy, nursing, medicine preferably rehabilitation medicine), psychology and social work. Advice from a psychiatrist, teacher, careers adviser and orthotist should also be available. Treatment, too, requires team work, preferably from a team that not only works towards the same goals but also shares approaches to treatment and accepts overlapping professional roles [10]. Why is this so important in TBI rehabilitation? There are two main reasons.

- Physical, cognitive and emotional problems virtually never occur in isolation. Instead they not only tend to occur together but also interact. If viewed from only one perspective, problems might be misconstrued.
- Two of the overriding problems in TBI are poor memory and an impaired ability to generalize skills learned in a particular environment. If any new skill can be taught and reinforced in several different environments, perhaps with variations in approach, the chances that the patient will remember and be able to apply the new skill generally should theoretically improve.

THE EARLY PHASE.

Coma stimulation programmes

Both relatives and hospital staff tend to feel helpless when confronted by persistent coma; perhaps this is what has inspired the development of coma stimulation programmes. There are two schools of thought about the efficacy of such programmes. One school argues that cortical arousal depends partly on environmental stimulation and cites evidence that coma stimulation programmes may shorten the duration of coma [11]. The other school argues that the evidence is mainly anecdotal or drawn from very small trials and that certain forms of stimulation might lead to habituation and make matters worse [12]. While these arguments remain unresolved, it makes sense to administer any stimulation programme in a quiet environment, where background stimulation will not cause distraction. Indeed it is reasonable to assume that the severely brain-injured individual will have lost the ability to pay selective attention – to concentrate on relevant information – an ability crucial to learning [12].

It is also reasonable to assume that 'selective attention', if it exists in a particular individual, is likely to be short-lived. Each 'stimulation' session should, therefore, also be of short duration. How short, though? It is surprising that, although this requirement is widely acknowledged, some published coma stimulation programmes advise administering stimuli repeatedly via each of the sensory modalities. Such a sequence of stimulation would take approximately an hour to complete [12].

Anyone who has experience of working with severely affected conscious individuals will appreciate that such patients often have a concentration span of less than 15 minutes (indeed, sometimes fleeting). It makes little sense to administer stimuli to an unconscious patient for longer than this without a break. It is also important to appreciate that any stimulus to a patient (whether intended or not) must be regarded as such, whether it is administered as part of a coma stimulation programme or, perhaps, routine nursing care. Thus, coma stimulation cannot go on while the patient is turned in bed or a nurse pops her head round the door and says 'Hello'. Clearly, such a stimulus-regulated environment is very difficult to create in a busy ward.

Sensitivity to the needs and wishes of relatives and friends is important in all cases, but perhaps particularly so when the victim is in coma. Indeed, hospital staff are likely to find themselves the butt of angry relatives unless they anticipate their special needs [13]. On the basis of present evidence and given finite resources, it is difficult to set up theoretically appropriate programmes. It would also be difficult to justify coma stimulation programmes for all patients. However, the author's view is that relatives should be encouraged to follow a specified programme of stimulation, provided they understand the paucity of evidence for efficacy. This role may help stem their frustration.

They should also be encouraged to keep a diary of events in hospital. This serves several useful functions. As well as providing a further role, it helps both the rehabilitation team and the patient to subsequently fill in the gaps in information. The former may, for example, use the record to determine the duration of post-traumatic amnesia, while patients themselves often say that they feel less vulnerable once they know a little more of what happened while they were unconscious.

Fits and post-traumatic epilepsy

Fits occur with relative frequency in the first week following moderate or severe head injuries. These should not be termed epilepsy, although they are associated with an increased (25%) risk of subsequent post-traumatic epilepsy [14]. Prophylactic anticonvulsants may be prescribed. These may reduce the incidence of early fits [15], but their value as prophylaxis against later fits is controversial [15,16]. If anticonvulsants are to be used, it would be rational to confine their use to patients whose initial injury was complicated by:

- early fits;
- intracranial haematoma requiring evacuation;
- depressed fracture.

With these features the risks of developing post-traumatic epilepsy are 25%, 31% and 15% respectively, whereas without these the risk is only 1%, equivalent to that of the general population [14].

Carbamazepine and sodium valproate are better choices as anticonvulsants than phenytoin; the latter is less effective at controlling partial seizures and temporal lobe fits, both of which are seen with relative frequency after TBI. Also, though all have adverse effects, phenytoin appears to produce more marked depression of cognitive function [17], thus aggravating a problem which may already have been affected by the head injury itself.

In the early phases of rehabilitation, seizures may have little impact on functional recovery; they are important when return to work and/or driving are considered and are therefore discussed later.

Movement disorders

Following TBI two main types of movement disorder are seen: loss of mobility – usually hemiparesis or quadraparesis – and involuntary movement.

In contrast to coma stimulation and prophylactic anticonvulsants, there is no doubt about the efficacy of available strategies to prevent the secondary consequences of immobility: pressure sores and contractures. Nevertheless, such sequelae occur commonly. For example, in a point prevalence study carried out in a large teaching hospital in 1989, over 5% of all in-patients had pressure sores [18] while another survey of 58 head-injured patients who were being cared for in general wards in a teaching hospital identified 12 patients with contractures [19]. Strategies for the prevention of these problems are described below. The general principles to be followed to avoid pressure sores are summarized in Table 9.2.

Table 9.2 Pressure sores – risk factors and methods of reducing these

Risk factors	Strategies to reduce these

Pressure = $\dfrac{\text{weight}}{\text{area}}$	1. Reduce obesity
	2. Increase weightbearing area by
	  a) calorie supplementation if underweight
	  b) using compliant (e.g. foam), flowing (e.g. air, gels) or rigid, moulded (e.g. rigid plastics, vacuum-moulded cushions) materials

Quality of skin poor	1. Improve perfusion; treat hypotension aggressively 2. Improve nutrition; dietary supplements treat additional medical problems, e.g. infection 3. Treat incontinence
Rise in temperature	Allow air circulation and thus evaporation to cool skin, e.g. use mattresses that circulate air
Shear	Use additional layer to take up shear when moving patient, e.g. draw sheet.
Time spent on a given area	1. Regular moving/turning of patient (often impractical; requires high staffing levels; useful for conscious, motivated patients) 2. Use of mattress with channels that are inflated alternately and thus alternate areas of skin contact

As indicated above, contractures frequently hamper rehabilitation efforts. Two factors contribute to their development: immobility and abnormal posture. The second of these may arise as a consequence of spasticity. Thus, efforts to reduce tone at an early stage in treatment by

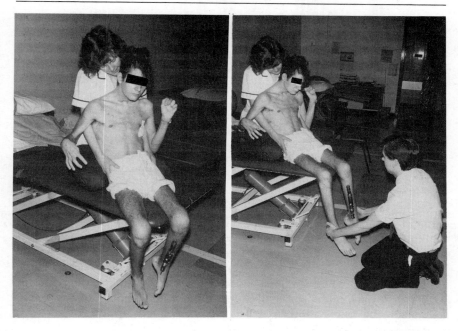

Figure 9.1 A patient receiving physiotherapy for joint contractures acquired through immobility.

physiotherapy, including careful movement and positioning of the joints and, if necessary, using medication is worthwhile. Figure 9.1 shows the development of contractures in a young man.

The first photo was taken shortly after he first recovered consciousness. However, he required a further period of assisted ventilation as a consequence of recurrent bilateral pneumothoraces, having sustained severe chest injuries in his initial road traffic accident. The contractures developed during this second period of intensive care treatment.

Although the contractures shown in these photos might have been avoidable, all the currently available techniques to minimize spasticity and reduce the incidence of contractures have certain disadvantages. For example, physiotherapy may be difficult or ineffective in a patient who is confused and/or in pain. Under these circumstances, the patient may not allow the physiotherapist to move or position a joint appropriately. In confused patients, a clear explanation of the purpose of any treatment session may enhance cooperation. Where pain exists, it is worth trying to time analgesia so that its effect is maximal during physiotherapy sessions. If hyperaesthesia is a problem, carbamazepine, of proven value in other types of neurogenic pain such as diabetic peripheral neuropathy, can be used.

Splinting joints to maintain position is a controversial subject. Some believe that splinting can make spasticity worse by stimulating the skin and triggering abnormal movement patterns. Others believe, on theoretical, neurophysiological grounds, that this would only occur with intermittent contact, not the maintained contact provided by a splint. There is little scientific data to confirm or refute these ideas. Two facts about orthoses are, however, indisputable. Firstly, rigid splinting requires skill in application if pressure sores over bony prominences are to be avoided. Secondly, a soft or flexible splint, which cannot maintain its own shape when counteracting a joint movement is, by definition, of little value, except perhaps as a visual and tactile reminder to the patient and others of where a joint should be positioned.

Medication has its drawbacks. Our own practice is to try a gradually increasing dose of a muscle relaxant such as baclofen or dantrolene, as both have dose-related side effects. Drowsiness, which would interfere with rehabilitation, and deteriorating control of continence are particularly relevant. Moreover, certain patients are dependent on a degree of spasticity for activities such as transfers via standing, so, for example, it may prove impossible to control upper limb spasm without losing useful lower limb spasm. A coordinated approach between therapist and doctor is, therefore, essential.

One useful therapeutic advance has been the introduction of techniques which localize the effects of the agent used to relax the muscle. Botulinum toxin has been used successfully in this way. It is expensive and its effects only last a few months, but is worth considering. Other alternatives are intrathecal baclofen, morphine or midazolam. These require skilled administration and are generally only suitable for paraplegia [20].

Myositis ossificans sometimes develops around contracted or immobile joints. Fortunately, this painful condition is relatively rare. The antecedents may either be local injury in the initial accident or local injury during over-vigorous mobilization. Either might cause muscle contusions that subsequently ossify [21]. The condition is best avoided by ensuring that mobilization is gentle and concentrates on active movement for, although various remedies have been tried, none have been particularly successful [22].

Movement disorders such as ataxia are difficult to treat. Drug treatment is usually disappointing, although beta-blockers may be worth a trial [23]. Stereotactic surgery may be an option in intractable problems but generally all that can be done is to stabilize the trunk using supportive seating while activities that depend on upper limb coordination are carried out. Sadly, even this can prove of little help; severe upper limb ataxia can prevent someone from feeding him/herself even though he/she may be able to walk. Generally the rehabilitation of hemiparesis following TBI yields good results, provided the strategies described above to prevent contractures, control tone and restore posture are adhered to and active exercises are encouraged to improve stamina. Nevertheless, the impact of even a minor residual motor disability can be considerable, bearing in mind prior abilities and expectations of this typically young group of patients.

Rehabilitation of communication and swallowing problems

Communication problems are covered in Chapter 15, where the authors describe their own experience of using group therapy to enhance communication skills in patients many months after the initial injury.

Swallowing problems, on the other hand, often need to be addressed very early in a rehabilitation programme, for if overlooked they can lead to inhalation pneumonia or malnutrition. The following questions need to be answered.

- Can all consistencies of food or drink be safely swallowed? If not, are certain consistencies safe e.g. semi-solids? A video fluoroscopy may help to establish this.
- Is oral calorie intake sufficient to maintain weight? If the answer to either of these questions is no, gastrostomy feeding is preferable to either nasogastric or intravenous feeding as a longer-term option [24].

The establishment of continence

The causes of incontinence following TBI are many. They can range from disruption of the neurological pathways that control sphincters, problems with mobility or orientation such that the patient cannot get himself to the toilet when necessary, to emotional problems such as disinhibition. The author has also encountered a patient whose constant demands for drinks and assistance to go to the toilet were attributed to behavioural problems following TBI. Further investigations revealed that this patient was unable to concentrate his urine because of hypothalamic damage causing diabetes insipidus.

This is exceptional. Generally, continence can be restored by first verifying that the patient is able to indicate need. (This may involve establishing a way of rapidly and reliably summoning help for a patient with communication and mobility problems.) Thereafter, the patient is encouraged to adhere to a regime of regular toileting. Oxybutinin and other anticholinergic drugs are occasionally used but are seldom necessary.

THE TRANSITIONAL PHASE

Rehabilitation of cognitive and emotional problems

Whereas disorders of movement, speech or continence tend to frustrate and depress patients, the significance of perceptual and other cognitive problems is seldom appreciated either by the patients themselves or by their relatives. Yet it is these, and also emotional problems, that account for much long-term handicap [25]. All too often, such problems only emerge when a patient returns home or attempts to return to work. Chapter 6 describes a community-based study to identify such problems in patients discharged from a regional neurosurgical unit, and highlights this point.

Is it possible to tackle cognitive and emotional problems prior to discharge into the community? There are certainly strong grounds for arguing that the problems should have been identified in hospital. An early screen to establish their nature and extent is a prerequisite for successful rehabilitation. Although poor memory and difficulty maintaining attention and concentration are characteristic features of severe head injury, these may be compounded by perceptual or receptive communication difficulties. Each difficulty could manifest in many different ways. For example, someone with an attentional disorder might respond with anger if his/her fragile concentration is broken by an unwanted and irrelevant distraction.

The rehabilitation unit is a convenient and safe environment to try out potential treatment programmes, although definitive management may be often impractical or ineffective in this environment. Typically, the head-injured person is able to learn new information and skills but is then unable to apply the new skills generally. Possibly this is due to placing undue reliance on implicit (non-conscious) memory (which tends to be situation-specific) because of impairment of explicit (conscious) memory systems [26]. The practical result is that what is learned in hospital, for example, is not continued at home.

To some extent a home environment can be simulated in hospital. In our own unit we use an assessment flat for this purpose. This may work well for those with minor or moderate difficulties, but is of limited value for those with very severe cognitive or behavioural problems. Thus, as described in Chapter 12, behaviour modification techniques can be very successful in a closely structured environment, where all interactions with the patient are carefully monitored. The challenge is either to reproduce the same situation at home or to generalize the behaviour to other varied environments.

Some have tackled this problem of generalization by using 'cognitive behaviour modification'. This technique is based on work with schizophrenics in the 1970s and 1980s [27]. It aims to increase insight and awareness through structured interviews.

The choice of approach must be influenced by the severity of patients' problems. Where cognition is so severely impaired that sufficient insight is impossible to achieve, the rehabilitation process will depend largely on techniques such as those described in Chapter 12.

However, for the less severely affected individual, a cognitive behaviour modification programme has the attraction that it seeks to allow the brain-injured individual to make an informed choice about his/her behaviour, rather than impose a code of behaviour on him/her. Retention and generalization should theoretically occur more readily, since learning a new code of behaviour in this way would depend on a higher level of processing (Chapters 10 and 11). Another approach, so far under-evaluated, is individual psychotherapy [28]. The authors point out that the therapist must work within the context of the life problem that brings the patient into therapy and the approach may need to be more direct, structured and innovative than with non-brain-injured individuals. It is particularly important for the therapist to appreciate the limitations imposed by a patient's cognitive deficits. (The therapist often has to be extraordinarily patient, persistent and innovative, yet firm and cheerful!)

Finally, Peters et al. [29] have described a pragmatic approach to behaviour modification designed to achieve community re-entry. Relatives, carers and others were enlisted, not only to help with behaviour modification, but also to ensure that goals were shared and feasible – agreed standards of acceptable behaviour. Failure to agree on goals has, in the authors' experience, led to the demise of many well-intentioned attempts to modify behaviour within the rehabilitation unit.

In chapters 10 and 11 the authors have used their understanding of slow information processing and memory impairment to derive general rules and encouraged their patients to apply these in differing settings. In Chapters 14 and 15 group therapy and role play have been used as means of simulating the real world more closely. Interestingly, these situations encouraged some patients to appreciate and express emotional feelings about their disabilities – something which might otherwise have been deferred till the patient went home and help was less readily available.

In our own unit we have tried one further approach – the use of a key worker to encourage a family to adopt, within their home, standard strategies to manage aggression in a very severely injured patient. We had previously found these strategies successful in hospital.

Good management of the transitional phase of rehabilitation should include a practical appraisal of day-to-day needs. This must be done prior to discharge from the rehabilitation unit and will normally involve discussion with relatives and other carers (both voluntary and those available from local health or social services). A home visit, usually carried out by an occupational therapist, will identify environmental alterations that are required.

COMMUNITY PHASE

There is sometimes a tendency to regard this as a static phase in which no further rehabilitation input is required. For most patients, particularly children and young adults this is inappropriate, for it is in this phase that many patients face their most difficult challenges. The transition from living with parents to living independently can be particularly hard. Few appreciate how much their life has been altered by their head injury until they try to return to their former lifestyle and find themselves confronted with obstacles. Often, this is when the grieving process begins and when counselling and support are needed most.

Stress may be increased by anxieties about legal matters; this sometimes seems to have a paralysing effect on recovery since many patients believe, wrongly, that their case for compensation will be weakened by recovery. In fact, when submitting a report in support of a claim for compensation, the doctor's (or other professional's) responsibility is to describe the disabilities and handicaps, discuss the potential for further recovery (or deterioration) and discuss the extent to which these problems are attributable to the accident. There is, thus, little to be gained from failing to achieve potential. Instead, being able to quantify the needs, e.g. for special equipment to pursue a new career, carries distinct advantages.

Unexpected practical difficulties may emerge. The head-injured person may find that he is legally barred from driving, yet this was previously his main form of transport. (The UK legal requirements are shown in Table 9.3.) He may also experience financial difficulties, perhaps because of unemployment.

Table 9.3 Eligibility for driving after serious head injury (these criteria do not apply for HGV driving)

Clinical features	Requirements
Fits more than 24 hours after injury	1 year off driving after most recent fit
Surgery – burr holes only	6 months off driving
Surgery – craniotomy	1 year off driving
Dural tear	1 year off driving
Early focal neurological signs and PTA > 24 h	6 months off driving
Visual loss or inattention	Barred from driving unless 120° horizontal vision plus 20° above and below this throughout horizontal range
Diplopia	Must be controlled by patch or glasses
Other perceptual cognitive or emotional problems	Depends on impact of these problems – inform DVLA

There may be practical solutions to these problems. In Britain, driving assessment can provide invaluable information not only on an individual's eligibility to drive but also on suitable vehicles and vehicle adaptations for those drivers or passengers who are left with physical disability (see list of useful addresses below).

Vocational assessments are also available, both via statutory services and the independent sector; these can advise on training and employment and should also be able to tailor their advice to meet individual interests and local job opportunities.

EFFECTS OF TBI ON THE VICTIM AND HIS/HER FAMILY OR CARER(S)

Initially, friends or relatives are likely to be numbed by the shock of the accident and may then find themselves on an emotional pendulum for many weeks. In this state, much information given to them may be poorly retained or misunderstood while chance, perhaps flippant, remarks might be given undue importance. At this stage it is, therefore, important to ensure that only consistent and reliable information is given, preferably by a clinical or rehabilitation team member identified as such to the family and friends. In Britain, several useful handbooks are available, particularly from voluntary organizations such as Headway; these are often appreciated. In Chapter 13, Michael Oddy discusses how families can be helped to adjust to their brain-injured relative.

For the patient, a period of unconsciousness followed by post-traumatic amnesia inevitably has certain psychological consequences. The patient's first recollection may, for example, be of being washed by someone he/she doesn't recognize, someone who, nevertheless, obviously knows him/her well and treats him/her in a familiar way. This may be followed by a few weeks of recovery on an acute ward where, for example, bodily functions are discussed openly and intimate handling by nursing and therapy staff are the norm. Yet the patient, who is confused about whom he/she has or hasn't met before and who doesn't want to appear unfriendly, is at risk of being labelled as disinhibited if he/she greets all and sundry with the same familiarity as shown to him/her. Furthermore, the patient may have spent several weeks learning that he/she was very ill and should therefore let others help. However, as rehabilitation begins, the patient is then encouraged to do as much as possible for him/herself. Unless this is accompanied by an explanation that he/she is no longer ill, a combination of anxiety and resentment is perhaps inevitable.

Finally, like his/her family or friends, the person who has suffered the TBI needs to grieve his/her loss. The anger, bitterness, guilt, depression, etc. that are all part of that grief may well manifest many months after the family or friends have recovered, since grief can only arise from a recognition of what has been lost. This stage needs to be anticipated, particularly as rehabilitation progresses, for it is necessary to make someone aware of their disabilities in order to help them overcome them. It is likely that some of the problems attributed to brain damage, such as poor motivation, are in fact a manifestation of depression in some patients.

CONCLUSION

In this chapter I have described the patterns of brain damage in severe head injury and discussed some of the impairments, disabilities and handicaps that may arise as a consequence. The following chapters describe ways of dealing with these. In each case, authors have drawn on their own experience.

Inevitably, when shared features are described, there is a tendency to gloss over the differences. Perhaps this is acceptable, if it enables one to develop some confidence when dealing with the very difficult problems presented by TBI. However, there is always the danger that, in attempting to define treatment for the typical patient, individual goals are ignored and society's norms are instead used as goals.

The rehabilitation team must continue to see the reduction of handicap as its aim, but not at the expense of individuality. Trying to strike a balance between these conflicting aims is one of the most difficult and most interesting problems in head injury rehabilitation.

USEFUL ADDRESSES

Headway, National Head Injuries Association, 7 King Edward Court, King Edward Street, Nottingham, NG1 1EW.
Banstead Mobility Centre, Damson Way, Orchard Hill, Queen Mary's Avenue, Carshalton, Surrey, SM5 4NR.

REFERENCES

1. Holbourn AHS. Mechanics of head injuries. *Lancet* 1943; ii: 438–441.
2. Chestnut RM, Marshall LF, Klauber MR *et al*. The role of secondary brain injury in determining the outcome of severe TBI. *Journal of Trauma* 1993; **34**(2): 216–222.
3. Ruff RM, Marshall LF, Crouch J *et al*. Predictors of outcome following severe head trauma: follow-up data from the Traumatic Coma Data Bank. *Brain Injury* 1993; **7**(2): 101–111.
4. Levin HS, Meyer CA, Grossman RG *et al*. Ventricular enlargement after closed head injury. *Archives of Neurology* 1981; **38**: 623–629.
5. Gudeman SK, Kishore PRS, Becker DP *et al*. Computed tomography in the evaluation of incidence and significance of post-traumatic hydrocephalus. *Radiology* 1981; **141**: 397–402.

6. Snoek J, Jennett B, Adams JH *et al*. Computerised tomography after recent severe head injury in patients without acute intracranial haematoma. *Journal of Neurology, Neurosurgery, and Psychiatry* 1979; **42**: 215–225.
7. Graham DI. *How reversible is the damage?* Abstracts, International Brain Forum, Oxford, 1993: 10.
8. Wilson JTL, Wiedmann KD, Hadley DM *et al*. Early and late MRI and neuropsychological outcome after head injury. *Journal of Neurology, Neurosurgery, and Psychiatry* 1988; **51**: 391–396.
9. Klauber MR, Marshall LF, Luerssen TG *et al*. Determinants of head injury mortality: importance of the low risk patient. *Neurosurgery* 1989; **24**(1): 31–36.
10. Finset A. Subacute brain injury rehabilitation: a program description and a study of staff program evaluation. *Scandinavian Journal of Rehabilitation Medicine* 1992; **26**(Suppl): 25–33.
11. Mitchell S, Bradley VA, Welch JL *et al*. Coma arousal procedure: a therapeutic intervention in the treatment of head injury. *Brain Injury* 1990; **4**: 273–279.
12. Wood RL. Critical analysis of the concept of sensory stimulation for patients in vegetative states. *Brain Injury*, 1991; **5**: 401–409.
13. Stern JM, Sazbon L, Becker E *et al*. Severe behaviour disturbance in families of patients with prolonged coma. *Brain Injury* 1988; **2**(3): 259–262.
14. Jennett B. *Epilepsy After Non-missile Head Injuries*. London: Heinemann, 1975.
15. Temkin NR, Dikmen SS, Wilensky AJ *et al*. A randomised double-blind study of phenytoin for the prevention of post-traumatic epilepsy. *New England Journal of Medicine* 1990; **323**: 497–502.
16. Soroker N, Groswasser Z, Costeff H. Practice of prophylactic anticonvulsant treatment in head injury. *Brain Injury* 1989; **3**(2): 137–140.
17. Trimble MR. Anticonvulsant drugs and cognitive function: a review of the literature. *Epilepsia* 1987; **28**(Suppl 3): 537–545.
18. Crosier L. Personal communication.
19. Wilson BA, Shiel A, Watson N *et al*. Monitoring behaviour during coma and post traumatic amnesia. In: Christensen, Uzzell B, eds. *Progress in the Rehabilitation of Brain-injured People*. Hillsdale NJ: Lawrence Erlbaum Associates, (in press).
20. Siegfried J, Rea GL. Intrathecal application of drugs for muscle hypertonia. *Scandinavian Journal of Rehabilitation Medicine* 1988; **Suppl 17**: 145–148.
21. Booth DW, Westers BM. The management of athletes with myositis ossificans traumatica. *Canadian Journal of Sports Sciences* 1989; **14**: 10–16.
22. Bruni L, Giammaria P, Tozzi MC *et al*. Fibrodysplasia ossificans progressiva. An 11 year-old boy treated with a diphosphonate. *Acta Paediatrica Scandinavica*, 1990; **79**: 994–998.
23. Ellison PH. Propranolol for severe post-head injury action tremor. *Neurology* 1978; **28**: 197–199.
24. Hull MA, Rawlings J, Murray FE *et al*. Audit of outcome of long-term enteral nutrition by percutaneous endoscopic gastrostomy. *Lancet* 1993; **341** (8849): 869–872.
25. Brooks DN, McKinlay W, Symington C *et al*. Return to work within the first seven years of severe head injury. *Brain Injury* 1987; **1**: 5–19.
26. McAndrews MP, Glitsky E, Schacter DL. When priming persists: long-lasting implicit memory for a single episode in amnesic patients. *Neuropsychologia*, 1987; **25**(3): 497–506.

27. Cameron R, Meichenbaum D. Cognition and behaviour change. *Australian and New Zealand Journal of Psychiatry* 1980; **14**(2): 121–125.
28. Carberry H, Burd B. Individual psychotherapy with the brain injured adult. *Cognitive-Rehabilitation* 1986; **4**(4): 22–24.
29. Peters MD, Gluck M, McCormick M. Behaviour rehabilitation of the challenging client in less restrictive settings. *Brain Injury* 1992; **6**(4): 299–314.

Evaluation of memory rehabilitation:

many questions and some answers

10

Ina J. Berg, Betto G. Deelman and
Marthe Koning-Haanstra

INTRODUCTION

In clinical practice, as well as in scientific research, a therapist trying to evaluate the effectiveness of memory rehabilitation is confronted with many questions. In this chapter we will shortly discuss some of the most important issues (whom to treat, what to treat, how to treat and how to know if a treatment has been sensible) and for each topic describe the choices we made in our evaluation study on memory strategy training.

AIMS OF TREATMENT

As in rehabilitation in general, in memory therapy it is essential to explicitly formulate treatment goals [1,2]. Before treatment starts these goals ought to be clear both to the therapist and to the subject. In memory therapy one can broadly distinguish three classes of goal [3].

- **Improving memory**: Here one can think of ambitious goals such as 'improve your memory' or even 'prevent dementia', slogans used by commercial memory schools and in advertisements for memory medicines. By now, it is widely acknowledged that it is impossible to restore memory capacity once lost by neurological damage or normal ageing. With restoration beyond the scope of rehabilitation, one should instead concentrate on amelioration: teaching subjects to make a more efficient use of remaining capacities. We believe the goals for memory treatment have to be limited to improvement of performance in specific memory domains. The narrower goal of 'improving the ability of the patient to remember appointments' seems far more realistic and far more measurable than the general restoration aims.

- **Reducing memory complaints and anxiety**: There are several possible methods achieving a reduction in complaints and anxiety related to memory failures. One is to explain to the subject how memory works and how memory can be affected by brain damage or ageing. If the subject learns to understand and accept these changes, anxiety and concern may decrease. Within this class of goals, memory performance is of secondary concern. If one succeeds in reducing anxiety, it is conceivable (but by no means guaranteed) that through reduced tension memory performance may increase.
- **Improving prerequisites for memory**: There are some patients whose memory deficits are a direct consequence of underlying problems, e.g. attention or concentration deficits. Here again one does not tackle memory problems directly, but indirectly by treating supposedly underlying causes, e.g. by attention or concentration training or perception exercises. Whether this is appropriate for a given subject will have to become clear from a thorough assessment of functional deficits.

Of course there is overlap in goals. The point to be made here is that one should carefully consider what the main goals of treatment are, since these will have consequences for the method of treatment, expectation of results and, very importantly, evaluation requirements.

In our study we chose memory performance improvement as an aim and we let the patients determine the specific targets of the treatment. In a problem analysis, they had to indicate which memory problems were most distressing for them in daily life and thus had to be dealt with in the training. In this way the therapeutic programme was individualized to a high degree, ensuring that it was relevant to the patient and that he/she was motivated to continue with it. On average, three problems were treated per patient. An overview of the frequencies of the treated problems can be seen in Table 10.1.

As shown in the table, there are a number of very common problems in our patient group – forgetting names or forgetting because of lack of concentration – but we also treated some rather idiosyncratic problems.

METHODS OF COGNITIVE REHABILITATION

Even when the aim of treatment is restricted to teaching a subject to make more efficient use of his/her remaining memory capacities, there are still many methods of trying to achieve this. One of the choices to

Table 10.1 Complaints treated in the strategy training condition – no. and percentage of CHI patients for whom these were the targets of training

Complaint	n	%
Forgetting peoples' names	14	82
Forgetting due to distractibility	11	65
Forgetting written texts	7	41
Forgetting conversations	6	35
Forgetting routes/getting lost	4	24
Forgetting timing of events	3	18
Commands for computer program	1	6
Composition of samples for chemical analyses	1	6
Medical terminology	1	6
Forgetting to write down appointments	1	6
Straying from the subject	1	6
Forgetting customer and complaint	1	6

be made is between group or individual treatment. Both forms have their own specific advantages. In a group, group members can learn from each other. They can be reassured by finding that others have the same problems (but perhaps be shocked to learn that they have the worst) and being in a group can clearly have some social advantages. On the other hand, it is very hard for a therapist in a group to adjust the treatment to individual needs, strengths and preferences. These restrictions of group treatment are essentially the plus-points of individual treatment. In practice, the choice for group sessions is often made for time- and money-saving reasons, but it would seem advisable to make a cost–benefit analysis. It might turn out that a few hours of individual guidance is as effective as weeks of group therapy.

Whether one chooses group or individual therapy, many treatment methods are possible, the choice probably largely depending on the problem and, of course, the subject(s). Again, it is possible to distinguish three classes.

- **External devices**: for some memory problems it seems most appropriate to advise external memory aids, such as diaries, notebooks, calendars or even electronic diaries [4]. Teaching an efficient use of these aids encompasses bringing system in to the notes and regularity in the times these are consulted, possibly with the use of another external aid – an alarm-clock. Although this may seem easy for regular users of external aids (as most readers will be), for some subjects, e.g. densely amnesic patients, it appears to be very hard [5]. However, it seems sensible to at least try the use of external memory aids, if only to save effort. The patients in our study were always advised to use external aids for information that is easily written down or looked up.

- **Repetitive practice**: with a drill and practice approach (repeating a task over and over again), it is possible to teach most subjects a certain task. Sometimes this is just what is needed for a particular patient – for instance an institutionalized, demented patient may learn the route from the living room to the bathroom by repetitive practice – but mostly treatments are meant to generalize to other problem areas as well. Certainly, one cannot assume that repetitive practice stimulates memory in such a way that memory in general is strengthened as if it were a mental muscle [6,7]. Even if generalization is not aimed for, it seems that, though drill and practice can result in gains, 'the cost–benefit ratio is not supportive of using the method on a regular basis' [8]. In our study, we used the drill and practice method in a subgroup of patients as a control treatment ('pseudotraining'), from which no generalization effects were expected.
- **Internal strategies**: here we can make a distinction between the traditional pragmatic mnemonics (e.g. imagery, method of loci, peg-word system or keyword method) and the theoretical principles found by psychological memory researchers to help encoding and retrieval. Of the classical methods, advocated as early as 500 BC, imagery is most widely studied. It appeared to be more effective than no strategy for brain-damaged individuals to recall words [2,9–11], to recall paired associates [12–15] and to recall names [2,9,11]. However, some important conclusions have been drawn by the researchers that must have implications for the use of imagery in memory rehabilitation. Artificial mnemonics are rather difficult to learn, as was found by Cermak [15] in a group of Korsakoff patients, and require much effort and creativity in their application. Baddeley & Warrington [12] found that their amnesic patients were able to form images, but that they were not able to create interactive images. Even more important are the following results: Wilson [2] found that imagery, though effective for learning names, did not generalize, even to other names. Lewinsohn et al. [9] and Goldstein et al. [11] found that imagery was a more effective strategy for learning word-pairs than for much more relevant information in daily life: learning names of persons. Besides, in the study of Lewinsohn et al. [9] it appeared that the effects of imagery training did not generalize over time. The moderately positive effects of imagery training were no longer detectable in the 1-week follow-up, either in the patient group or in the normal control group. Though the other classic mnemonics have not been studied as extensively, one might assume that the method of loci, the peg-word system etc., all heavily relying on

interactive imagery, are even more difficult to learn, to retain and, especially, to apply in daily life.

To keep the motivation in our patients high and to stimulate actual application in daily life, we chose to teach the patients some more simple and easy to use strategies. In a booklet we translated relevant results of psychological memory research as a set of general 'memory rules' for laymen.

In this booklet, preceding the more concrete rules, some general recommendations are emphasized.

- **It is impossible to cure your memory**: that is, it is not possible to repair or exchange nerve cells and, so far, an effective 'memory pill' has not been produced. Yet you can make more efficient use of your remaining capacities. However, this takes time and effort.
- **Acceptance**: try to accept that your memory is impaired to a certain degree and let others accept this too. Only then is it possible to react calmly when an appeal is made on your memory and avoid frustration when you have forgotten something. Tension will only make your memory performance worse.
- **External Memory Aids**: use external aids whenever possible. Why try to learn things by heart when they can easily be written down or looked up? Then the more technical, specific memory rules are described. These are, briefly summarized.
- **Attention**: pay attention to the information to be remembered. Make sure that you are not distracted by your environment and that you consciously focus on what you have to remember.
- **Time**: give yourself more time to remember things. Generally, the more time you spend, the more you will remember. But spend your time economically – not too long without a pause, but frequently and little by little.
- **Repetition**: whatever you have to remember will sink in more easily if you repeat it, and there are several forms of repetition: simple repetition, spaced repetition (with increasing time intervals) and varied repetition (in several ways and situations).
- **Association**: making verbal associations (for example linking items together in a 'story') and/or forming visual images makes remembering easier.
- **Organization**: try to categorize or arrange the information to be remembered. For example, when you have to go shopping, try to group your purchases into groceries, dairy produce, vegetables, etc. and when you have to remember a text, try to identify the organization or structure.

- **Anticipation and Retrospection**: try to link the input and retrieval situations. When you know you'll need information in the future, try to anticipate the retrieval situation vividly and link input and retrieval. When you have to retrieve information you have stored in memory in the past, try to think back to the input situation.

In order to make remembering of the specific memory rules ('Attention' to 'Anticipation') easier, an example of a first-letter mnemonic is given. It is a short sentence, in which the words start with the initial letters of the memory rules, which are all different, at least in Dutch. Unfortunately, this is not directly translatable into English, but it says something like: 'when aunty coughs, our floor creaks'.

Finally, the importance of a systematic approach is brought up in the last recommendation.

- **Work in a systematic way**: whatever method you use to remember or retrieve information, try to use that method systematically.
  And, very important, try to arrange your own surroundings in a systematic way, so you do not have to search each time you need a particular item.

Treatment always began by discussing, explaining and, most importantly, demonstrating all these memory rules. The patient also received a workbook, in which he/she could write down the most important exercises and experiences with each particular memory rule. In this way the workbook became a personal memory book.

After the choice of training aims was made, training then consisted of both laboratory sessions and daily homework exercises. Though the specific approach of the training differed for each complaint and each patient, treatment always took place along established lines in four phases. The first phase consisted of a thorough complaint analysis, in which the patient and the therapist tried to find out when, how and why the specific memory problem occurred. In the second phase the most applicable memory rules were chosen from the booklet and explained. Practically, this meant different strategies were highlighted for different complaints. In the third phase these strategies were demonstrated and exercised with standard material. The fourth and most important phase in the strategy training was employing the learned strategies on material relevant to the patient in the laboratory sessions and in daily life situations as homework. A more detailed description of the therapy can be found in three case studies published by Deelman, Berg and Koning-Haanstra [16]. The treatment consisted of about 18 1-hour (three times a week for 6 weeks) individual sessions and about 18 hours of homework exercises, stressing the importance of applying the learned strategies in daily life.

SELECTION OF PATIENTS AND/OR CLIENTS

We think it is necessary to explicitly formulate exclusion criteria for every intervention, such as 'this programme is unsuitable for patients with a severe aphasia' or 'with a total lack of insight', etc. Even if these general criteria have been met by the subject, in rehabilitation it is very important to take into account the characteristics, strengths and weaknesses of each individual client or patient. The goals and methods of intervention can differ according to type of lesion, type of deficit or subjective problem(s), acute or chronic stage of the illness, age, educational level, social situation, etc. It is obvious that patients with verbal memory deficits have need of a different type of treatment from patients with a non-verbal memory deficit, the elderly have to be treated differently from younger subjects, and intelligence-impaired patients require a different approach from the bright and intelligent ones. It has been argued that therapy might be most effective if given when the brain is in the midst of recovery and might still be optimally sensitive for stimulation, but before the patient has had the opportunity to adopt inappropriate strategies. However, the drawback of an early intervention is that the patient may not even fully realize what his/her cognitive impairments are and how they will interfere with daily life and, as a consequence, not yet be motivated to engage in a demanding memory therapy [17].

The subjects chosen for our evaluation study were chronic closed-head-injury (CHI) patients. The symptomatology of chronic CHI patients is often restricted to memory deficits, attention and personality changes [18,19] and complaints of forgetfulness are the most frequently reported subjective sequelae [20–22]. It has been demonstrated that memory performance does not show significant recovery in a 2-year period [23] and even 10–15 years post-injury disorders of memory have been found [24,25]. Furthermore, numerous studies have found that subjective memory complaints do not decrease with time [26–28]. CHI patients, thus, seem to be a group for whom memory rehabilitation would be most welcome, even more so since most of the CHI patients are young adults with a long life before them.

We selected CHI patients according to the following criteria:

- they had to be between 18 and 60 years of age;
- they had to have sustained their closed head injury at least 9 months earlier;
- they had to have subjective memory complaints in everyday life;
- there had to be objective evidence of memory deficits;
- those with significant (pre- or post-traumatic) intellectual, aphasic, apraxic, agnosic or personality disturbances were excluded; these judgements were made by two experienced clinical neuropsychologists with the decisive criterion of whether the disturbances

would hamper the understanding and execution of training instructions;

- those with other neurological or psychiatric hospital admissions were also excluded. Of course, motivation to participate was a decisive factor.

The group thus gathered consisted of 39 patients, with a rather 'lean' symptomatology. None of the patients was institutionalized any more. Slightly more than half of them (54%) had resumed their former work or educational activities, albeit in most cases at a lower level. The patients were randomly assigned to the treatment (strategy training) or control conditions (pseudotraining and no treatment), which will be described later.

As would be hoped for with random assignment, there are no statistically significant differences in biographical or neurological variables between the three CHI groups (Table 10.2). They did not differ in age, level of education, IQ, length of post-traumatic amnesia (PTA) or time since injury.

Table 10.2 Mean demographic and neurological data of the patient groups (Mann–Whitney U- and T-tests: no differences between CHI groups). PTA = post-traumatic amnesia

	n	Age	Level of education	IQ	Duration of PTA (days)	Time since injury (years)
Strategy training	17	36	5.1	105	29	5.4
Pseudotraining	11	33	4.5	106	35	6.3
No treatment	11	35	4.5	103	37	6.8

As can be seen from the length of PTA (around 1 month), these patients were severely brain-injured and, in view of the time since injury (with a mean of 6 years), they could be considered as chronic cases in whom spontaneous recovery seemed rather improbable. They were no longer under medical supervision or treatment.

EVALUATION

We strongly advocate that every intervention is evaluated, whether to see if an individual patient improves (as in clinical settings, where a single-case approach might be the most suitable method) or to see if an experimental treatment works (particularly in scientific research, where a choice must be made for controlled single-case trials or a group comparison study). An important issue in this field is the choice of reliable evaluation measures. Of course, the choice of the evaluation instrument(s) largely depends on the aims of treatment. 'Improving name recall' is evaluated differently from 'reducing memory complaints'. Further questions are: should we ask the patient to rate the improvement or should we rather rely on a more or less independent judge; what kind of objective tests or tasks are good measures of treatment and generalization effects, or should we use a combination of measurements?

In our study, we used four types of evaluation measure.

- **Subjective judgements**: first, we asked the patients their opinion on the quality and efficacy of treatment, the Subjective Ratings. Second, we administered a Memory Questionnaire similar to that of Sunderland, Harris and Gleave [29]. In this questionnaire, estimations of how often 37 everyday memory problems occurred to the subject during the last few weeks were given by the subjects themselves and by a close relative on a seven-point scale ranging from 1 = never to 7 = always.
- **Control tasks**: memory training should not have an effect on, for instance the speed of information processing. If one should find an improvement in reaction time scores, this could be attributable to spontaneous recovery effects or general motivational aspects. The reaction time tasks we used were: (1) a four-choice reaction time task and (2) a distraction reaction time task, both yielding separate decision and movement times.
- **Control memory tasks**: the three memory tests under this heading have in common that it is hardly possible to improve performance by employing conscious strategies such as association, organization or linking. They thus should not be affected by strategy training. We used the following tasks: (1) Media Information Test (MIT), a forced-choice recognition test for public events from 1981–87; (2) Warrington's Recognition Memory Faces (RMF), a forced-choice recognition test for faces and (3) The News, an auditory recall test for quickly presented newsflashes. For recognition tests, it is improbable that even the most sophisticated strategy will help in recognizing facts or faces, since all retrieval cues are available during the test. To understand the use of news recall as a strategy-insensitive task, a bit more explanation is required. Although strategy training might teach the subjects to organize the heard information (attention as a memory rule is discussed in both strategy and pseudotraining and is therefore not a distinctive strategy), the pace at which the newsflashes are read hardly leaves room for organizational strategies.
- **Target memory tasks**: strategy training should generalize to memory tasks that were not exercised during therapy but that are

strategy-sensitive. Performance should improve if subjects, for example, organize the material or form associations. The tasks used here were: (1) the 15 Words Test (a Dutch version of Rey's auditory verbal learning task, yielding an acquisition and a 15 min delayed recall score); (2) the Face–Name Learning task (with an acquisition and a 30 min delayed recall score) and (3) the Shopping List Task (with again an acquisition and a 30 min delayed recall score). The way in which these three tasks are administered gives the patients the opportunity to apply strategies, e.g. the items are slowly presented and there is some study time in all three tasks.

Within the three classes of objective data, the scores were combined into a number of sum scores. To avoid weighting problems in the addition of scores due to differences in score ranges between tests, test scores were standardized before they were added. For every variable, z-scores were computed, based on the scores obtained at the baseline assessments of all patients. So, each resulting z-score can be conceived of as the number of standard deviations from the mean of the patients at baseline. Z-scores on the separate tests were then added to three classes of sum scores.

- **Control sum scores**: the four standardized reaction time measures were combined to deliver the Total Reaction Time. A Decision Time and a Movement Time could be derived by combining two subscores.
- **Control memory sum scores**: a Control Memory Sum Score was computed by adding the standardized scores on the MIT, RMF and The News.
- **Target memory sum scores**: an overall memory performance score (Target Memory Sum Score) was obtained by adding all six scores of the three target tests. An Acquisition Score was computed by adding the three separate acquisition scores; likewise a Delayed Recall Score was obtained. These three sum scores are considered the most crucial indices in determining the effect of strategy training.

The advantages of working with subscores are that they reduce the number of statistical tests needed and that makes it possible to examine the 'overall' effects of training. Besides, in our data, the retest reliabilities of the sum scores are considerably higher than those of the separate scores, which is of the utmost importance in evaluation studies.

Another topic in evaluation is the timespan of effectiveness: we should not be satisfied with a short-lived improvement (the difference from baseline to immediately after training). To check whether the patient benefits from the intervention for a longer period, at least a long-term follow-up assessment is necessary.

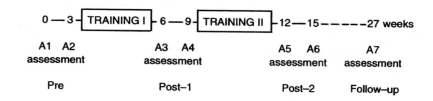

Figure 10.1 Study design.

All patients in our study were assessed seven times, according to the following time-schedule: during the first 3 weeks, two baseline assessments (A1 and A2) took place; the next 3 weeks were spent on the first training period, followed by two assessments (A3 and A4). The second training period was completed 3 weeks later and again was followed by two test sessions (A5 and A6). Finally, about a half year (27 weeks) after the start of the study (that is about 4 months after termination of therapy), a follow-up assessment took place (A7) (Figure 10.1).

To reduce the enormous amount of data and the individual variability in scores (causing 'noise', especially in individual and small group data), scores were pooled over the baseline period (A1–A2: Pre), the first post treatment period (A3–A4: Post-1), the second post treatment period (A5–A6: Post-2), and the long-term follow-up (A7: Follow-up). With these four time-points we could not only analyse the gain from baseline to follow-up (the most important difference), but also check if the changes were already visible earlier – that is, after the first and/or the second training period.

The last topics to be discussed are concerned with problems and possibilities in group comparison research. When analysing the effectiveness of a therapeutic programme, one needs to control for a number of alternative explanations of possible improvement, e.g. spontaneous recovery, motivational effects, retest effects and Hawthorne effects.

We controlled for **spontaneous recovery effects** in a number of ways: first by selecting only those patients who had sustained their injury at least 9 months previously (so spontaneous recovery would seem highly unlikely), by randomly assigning patients to three different treatment groups (so it would be very unlikely that one group should spontaneously recover more than the other groups) and by administering control tasks sensitive for non-specific effects (such as general recovery or general motivational improvement).

Retest effects were controlled for by adding a no-treatment group to the two treatment groups. This no-treatment group, of course, was assessed as often and with the same time intervals as the two treated groups. By group comparison one can thus eliminate the retest gains from the total gain made by the trained patients. Another often made suggestion to reduce retest effects is to use parallel versions of tests. Our experience with parallel versions (we actually used parallel versions for most of our tasks) is that they also show retest effects [30]. Possible explanations are, for example, the subject's growing familiarity with the testing situation and the test requirements, a decreased level of tension or the gradual development of an approach to tackling the task at hand.

Hawthorne effects (performing better as a result of receiving attention, for example, from a therapist) were controlled for by the group of pseudotreatment patients. These patients received the same amount of attention from a therapist and spent the same amount of time on memory games and exercises as the strategy group, but learned no strategies other than attention, time and simple repetition, the drill and practice method.

Finally, we think it is of the greatest importance to control for **individual differences** as well, especially in an heterogeneous population such as CHI patients and even more so in small group studies. We accounted for interindividual variability (besides by random group assignment) in a statistical, covariance-like way. A regression equation was used to determine the effects of the training methods while controlling statistically for interindividual differences in baseline performance. So, the post-treatment score was predicted from: (1) the baseline level of that score (PRE), (2) a dummy variable representing the strategy condition and (3) a dummy variable representing the pseudotraining condition.

On all measures, the baseline level was expected to be the best predictor of the later scores, but the question was whether the strategy and pseudotraining dummies could significantly contribute to the regression equation. In the following results, any significant change in proportion of variance explained by these dummies will be called 'effect'.

Table 10.3 Mean subjective ratings for the training (10-point scale ranging from 1 = lowest possible to 10 = highest possible)

	Strategy training mean	(range)	Pseudotraining mean	(range)
Satisfaction with the training	8	(6–10)	8	(7–10)
Personal fit of the training	8	(6–10)	8	(7–10)
Applicability in daily life	7	(3–9)	7	(6–8)
Recommendability to other patients	9	(6–10)	9	(7–10)

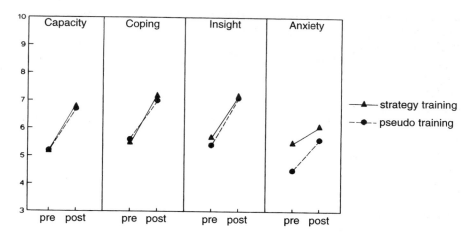

Figure 10.2 Subjective judgements of strategy training and pseudotraining. Mean subjective ratings before and after the training of the trained CHI groups (10-point scale, ranging from 1 = lowest possible to 10 = highest possible).

RESULTS

The main results of our evaluation study, then, are as follows:

- **Subjective judgements**: To put it mildly, the subjective data are not clearly in favour of the strategy training. The control patients were as highly satisfied with the treatment and the results of training as the strategy patients (Table 10.3 and Figure 10.2).

Also, with respect to other subjective data (Memory Questionnaire), there were no specific effects of strategy training. Even the no-treatment group reported less and less memory complaints in the course of the study. And these results are true for judgements of patients and relatives alike (Figure 10.3).

- **Control Sum Scores**: The mean scores for the three groups are depicted in Figure 10.4 and the results of the regression analyses are summarized in Table 10.4. After baseline level had been accounted for, no single effect of strategy training was found on the reaction time tasks, and the one significant contribution (post-2, movement time) to the regression equation of the pseudotraining cannot be conceived of as convincing evidence of rehabilitation effects.
- **Control Memory Sum Score**: Regression analyses showed that neither strategy training nor pseudotraining could add significantly to the equation once baseline level was accounted for, either at follow-up, post-2, or post-1 (Table 10.5 and Figure 10.5).

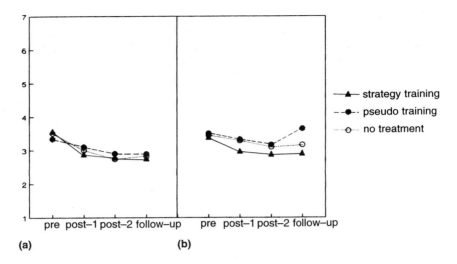

Figure 10.3 **(a)** Subjects' and **(b)** relatives' judgements of memory problems. Mean scores on the Memory Questionnaire by patients themselves and relatives. Non-parametric tests: within groups, significant changes over time in all groups; between groups, no significant differences.

- **Target Memory Sum Scores:** Summarizing the results of the regression analyses (Table 10.6 and Figure 10.6), baseline level was again the best predictor of post-treatment performance but, whereas not even a single significant effect of pseudotraining was found, strategy training appeared to have significant positive effects on all

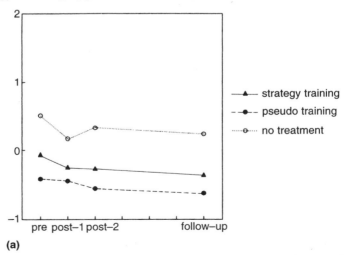

Figure 10.4 Standardized and combined scores on control tasks **(a)** Total Reaction Time.

three memory performance measures. These effects were strongest at follow-up, less prominent after the second training period and absent after the first 3 weeks of training. The table, furthermore, shows that the effects were strongest for Delayed Recall – in our view the most relevant measure for everyday life.

Summarizing, the results show that post-treatment test performance is best predicted by the level at which the subject performed prior to

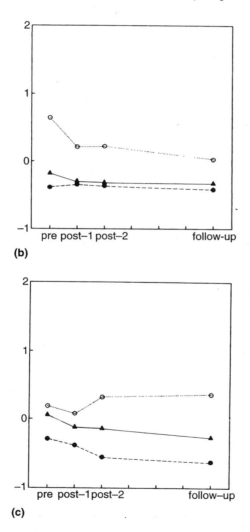

(b)

(c)

Figure 10.4 Standardized and combined scores on control tasks. **(b)** Decision Time. **(c)** Movement Time.

Table 10.4 Summarized results of regression analyses of the control tasks (significance two-tailed (*): $0.05 > p < 0.10$; *: $p \leqslant 0.05$; **: $p \leqslant 0.01$; ***: $p \leqslant 0.001$)

Criteria	Predictor	Baseline R^2	Strategy training R^2 change	Pseudotraining R^2 change
Post-1	Total reaction time	0.816***	0.000	0.000
	Decision time	0.814***	0.005	0.002
	Movement time	0.847***	0.001	0.000
Post-2	Total reaction time	0.827***	0.001	0.005
	Decision time	0.876***	0.002	0.000
	Movement time	0.734***	0.004	0.028*
Follow-up	Total reaction time	0.652***	0.001	0.001
	Decision time	0.571***	0.000	0.003
	Movement time	0.647***	0.009	0.014

treatment. Only the strategy condition yielded a significant positive extra effect on objective memory performance measures over and above this baseline effect.

Surprisingly, it appears that the largest effect of strategy training was found 4 months after therapy. This could be explained by the assumption that the subjects continued to practise the learned strategies in daily life and therefore performed better on the tasks at follow-up than immediately after training. However, we have no independent evidence for that, other than the remarks of patients at follow-up, which indicated that they still used the strategies they had learned during therapy.

It has to be pointed out that our treatment approach differs from most other programmes. Whereas our training is aimed at daily life situations and our evaluation is aimed at measuring generalization to 'standard' tests, most other treatments use strategies with standard laboratory material (e.g. word lists and word pairs), hoping for a generalization to daily life.

Teaching closed-head-injury patients to use strategies to overcome their individual daily problems thus seems to allow generalization to

Table 10.5 Summarized results of regression analyses of the control memory tasks (significance two-tailed (*): $0.05 > p < 0.10$; *: $p \leqslant 0.05$; **: $p \leqslant 0.01$; ***: $p \leqslant 0.001$)

Criteria	Predictor	Baseline R^2	Strategy training R^2 change	Pseudotraining R^2 change
Post-1	Control memory sum	0.816***	0.003	0.011
Post-2	Control memory sum	0.844***	0.014(*)	0.000
Follow-up	Control memory sum	0.732***	0.010	0.000

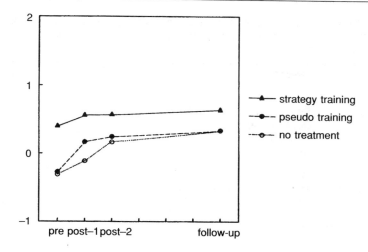

Figure 10.5 Standardized and combined score on control memory tasks.

tasks not specifically trained in the therapy. That this improvement on memory tasks is not due to effects of spontaneous recovery or to general motivational aspects can be deduced from the fact that strategy training does not result in better performance on the reaction time tasks or control memory tasks. Neither can it be due to Hawthorne effects, since pseudo-training does not result in significant gains.

Besides this hoped-for pattern, consisting on the one hand of improvement on strategy-sensitive tasks and on the other hand of no improvement on 'control' tasks, patients in the strategy condition also subjectively report an improvement in memory functioning. However, and this was not expected, the pseudotrained patients reported the same improvement in subjective wellbeing. As far as objective data are concerned, the pseudopatient group improved to the same degree as those who received no treatment but who are only repeatedly tested: the effect of drill and practice of memory tasks and games is certainly not larger than simple re-test effects.

The results on the group means very positively demonstrate a larger score increase in the strategy group than in the other two groups, but they do not say anything about individual performance changes. For clinicians, individual data will probably be more interesting. In determining which patients made a significant improvement from baseline to follow-up, we calculated the Reliable Change index (RC) [31], a recommendable criterion in single-case treatment evaluation for deciding whether a gain can be considered as significant. Table 10.7 shows the proportion of patients in the treated groups who made a significant improvement at a 5% level on the target memory sum scores.

Table 10.6 Summarized results of regression analyses of the target memory tasks (significance two-tailed (*): $0.05 > p < 0.10$; *: $p \leqslant 0.05$; **: $p \leqslant 0.01$; ***: $p \leqslant 0.001$)

Criteria	Predictor	Baseline R^2	Strategy training R^2 change	Pseudotraining R^2 change
Post-1	Memory sum	0.721***	0.006	0.000
	Acquisition	0.601***	0.001	0.004
	Delayed recall	0.758***	0.014(*)	0.004
Post-2	Memory sum	0.644***	0.025(*)	0.003
	Acquisition	0.593***	0.021(*)	0.001
	Delayed recall	0.656***	0.031*	0.008
Follow-up	Memory sum	0.657***	0.048*	0.000
	Acquisition	0.563***	0.037*	0.000
	Delayed recall	0.699***	0.055**	0.000

On all three measures there are considerably more strategy patients than pseudotreatment patients who improved significantly. The largest number of improvers in the strategy group is found on the delayed recall score, the most relevant measure for everyday life. In the pseudotreated group there are only two patients improving significantly – one of whom spontaneously told us he used associational strategies!

PREDICTION

The last topic we would like to discuss is prediction: what factors contribute to success of training and what factors are of no value. If one were

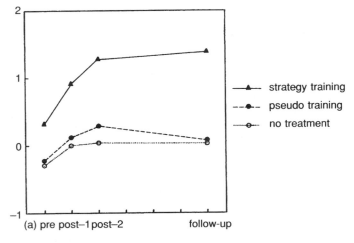

Figure 10.6 Standardized and combined scores on target memory tasks. **(a)** Target Memory Sum.

to find clear predictive variables, this could be important in deciding whether or not a patient would be a suitable candidate for therapy.

We again looked at the individual successful cases to see whether we could discover some common characteristics in these patients, but on the face of it, it appeared that the improvers represented the whole range of ages, educational levels, IQs, PTA lengths and times since injury. To make a more objective attempt at prediction, another regression analysis on the follow-up results was performed. To answer

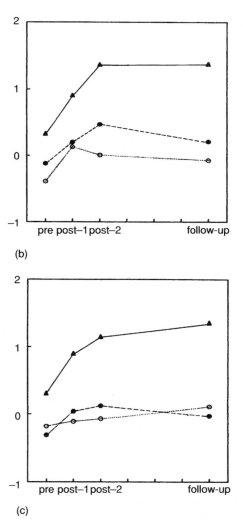

(b)

(c)

Figure 10.6 Standardized and combined scores on target memory tasks.   **(b)** Acquisition.   **(c)** Delayed Recall.

Table 10.7 Proportions (and percentages) of the patients in the treated groups who made a significant improvement at a 5% level on the target memory sum scores.

| | Strategy training | | Pseudotraining | |
	n	%	n	%
Memory sum	9/17	53	2/11	18
Acquisition	7/17	41	2/11	18
Delayed recall	12/17	71	2/11	1

questions such as 'is improvement of performance, irrespective of treatment, dependent on the severity of injury or demographic variables?', we entered the following variables in the equation as predictors: educational level and age and neurological factors such as the length of PTA and time since injury. As further predictors we added some interaction terms; i.e. baseline level, education, age, PTA and time since injury within the strategy condition. These were meant to answer questions like 'are younger patients more likely to profit from strategy training?'

Surprisingly, only one of those nine variables seems to have an additional effect, that is level of education within the strategy group, which suggests the more highly educated profit more from strategy training, whereas neurological factors or age (up to 60) do not have any predictive power. However, as we saw in the individual data, patients with lower educational attainments can profit from strategy training as well.

Practically, these results mean that no further selection criteria than the ones described earlier are needed to make a reasonable chance of achieving objective success with memory strategy training in CHI patients. More specifically, within the population of CHI patients in a general hospital such as ours, for around 30% of the chronic patients between 18 and 60 years of age our strategy training can be expected to be fruitful. There is, however, no reason to assume that CHI patients younger than 18 or older than 60 cannot profit from strategy training, as long as other neuropsychological functions or personality disorders do not stand in the way of understanding the strategies and their application.

As for cost–benefit analysis, we have made a rough estimation of the costs of our strategy therapy. A full-time therapist who spends 20 hours on training and 30 hours on preparation per patient can treat 34 patients in one year. With a Dutch psychologist's salary, our treatment would cost $1000–1500 per patient, rather cheap in comparison with many other therapies.

REFERENCES

1. Wilson BA. Memory therapy in practice. In: Wilson B A, Moffat N, eds. *Clinical Management of Memory Problems*. London: Croom Helm, 1984: pp 89–111.
2. Wilson B. *Rehabilitation of Memory*. New York: Guilford Press, 1987.
3. Koning-Haanstra M, Deelman BG, Berg IJ. Resultaten van geheugentraining. In: de Jongh AJCM, Langendoen MW, den Boogert HL *et al.*, eds. *Aspecten van geheugen–vitaliteitstraining*. Rotterdam: Stichting Bij- en Nascholingskursussen KVV, 1990: pp 15–29.
4. Harris JE. Methods of improving memory. In: Wilson BA, Moffat N, eds. *Clinical Management of Memory Problems*. London: Croom Helm, 1984: pp 46–62.
5. Davies ADM, Binks MG. Supporting the residual memory of a Korsakoff patient. *Behavioural Psychotherapy* 1983; **11**: 62–74.
6. Milner B, Corkin S, Teuber JL. Further analysis of the hippocampal amnesic syndrome: a 14-year follow-up study of HM. *Neuropsychologia* 1968; **6**: 215–234.
7. Brooks DN, Baddeley AD. What can amnesics learn? *Neuropsychologia* 1976; **14**: 111–122.
8. Franzen MD, Haut MW. The psychological treatment of memory impairment: a review of empirical studies. *Neuropsychological Review* 1991; **2**(1): 29–63.
9. Lewinsohn PM, Danaher BG, Kikel S. Visual imagery as a mnemonic aid for brain-injured persons. *Journal of Consulting and Clinical Psychology* 1977; **45**(5): 717–723.
10. Kovner R, Mattis S, Goldmeier E. A technique for promoting robust free recall in chronic organic amnesia. *Journal of Clinical Neuropsychology* 1983; **5**: 65–71.
11. Goldstein G, McCue M, Turner SM *et al.* An efficacy study of memory training for patients with closed-head injury. *Clinical Neuropsychologist* 1988; **2**(3): 251–259.
12. Baddeley AD, Warrington EK. Memory coding and amnesia. *Neuropsychologia* 1973; **11**: 159–165.
13. Jones MK. Imagery as a mnemonic aid after left temporal lobectomy: contrast between material-specific and generalised memory disorders. *Neuropsychologia* 1974; **12**: 21–30.
14. Jones-Gotman M, Milner B. Right temporal-lobe contribution to image-mediated verbal learning. *Neuropsychologia* 1978; **16**: 61–71.
15. Cermak LS. Improving retention in alcoholic Korsakoff patients. *Journal of Studies on Alcohol* 1980; **41**: 159–169.
16. Deelman BG, Berg IJ, Koning-Haanstra M. Memory strategies for closed head injured patients. Do lessons in cognitive psychology help? In: Wood RL, Fussey I, eds. *Cognitive Rehabilitation in Perspective*. London: Taylor & Francis, 1990: pp 117–144.
17. Miller E. *Recovery and Management of Neuropsychological Impairments*. New York: John Wiley & Sons, 1984.
18. Newcombe F. Rehabilitation in clinical neurology: neuropsychological aspects. In: Vinken PJ, Bruyn GW, Klawans HL, eds. *Handbook of Clinical Neurology*, vol 2, 46: Neurobehavioral Disorders. Amsterdam: Elsevier, 1985: pp 609–642.

19. van Zomeren AH, Saan RJ. Psychological and social sequelae of severe head injury. In: Braakman R, ed. *Handbook of Clinical Neurology*, vol 13: Head Injury. Amsterdam: Elsevier Science Publishers, 1990: pp 397–420.
20. Oddy M, Humphrey M, Uttley D. Subjective impairment and social recovery after closed head injury. *Journal of Neurology, Neurosurgery, and Psychiatry* 1978; **41**: 611–616.
21. Tyerman A, Humphrey, M. Changes in self-concept following severe head injury. *International Journal of Rehabilitation Research* 1984; **7**(1): 11–23.
22. Zomeren AH van, Burg W van den. Residual complaints of patients two years after severe head injury. *Journal of Neurology, Neurosurgery, and Psychiatry* 1985; **48**: 21–8.
23. Deelman BG, Saan RJ. Memory deficits: assessment and recovery. In: Deelman BG, Saan RJ, van Zomeren AH, eds. *Traumatic Brain Injury: Clinical, Social and Rehabilitational Aspects*. Lisse: Swets & Zeitlinger, 1990: pp 49–76.
24. Smith E. Influence of site of impact upon cognitive performance persisting long after severe closed head injury. *Journal of Neurology, Neurosurgery, and Psychiatry* 1974; **37**: 719–726.
25. Roberts AH. *Severe Accidental Head Injury*. London: McMillan, 1979.
26. Brooks DN, Aughton ME, Bond MR et al. Cognitive sequelae in relationship to early indices of severity of brain damage after severe blunt head injury. *Journal of Neurology, Neurosurgery, and Psychiatry* 1980; **43**: 529–534.
27. McKinlay WW, Brooks DN, Bond MR et al. The short-term outcome of severe blunt head injury as reported by relatives of the injured persons. *Journal of Neurology, Neurosurgery, and Psychiatry* 1981; **44**: 527–533.
28. Oddy M, Coughlan T, Tyerman A et al. Social adjustment after closed head injury: a further follow-up seven years after injury. *Journal of Neurology, Neurosurgery, and Psychiatry* 1985; **48**: 564–568.
29. Sunderland A, Harris JE, Gleave J. Memory failures in everyday life following severe head injury. *Journal of Clinical Neuropsychology* 1984; **6**: 127–142.
30. Berg IJ, Koning-Haanstra M, Deelman BG. Long-term effects of memory rehabilitation: a controlled study. *Neuropsychological Rehabilitation* 1991; **1**(2): 97–111.
31. Jacobson NS. Truax P. Clinical significance: A statistical approach to defining meaningful change in psychotherapy research. *Journal of Consulting and Clinical Psychology* 1991; **59**(1): 12–19.

Slow information processing and the use of compensatory strategies

11

Luciano Fasotti and Feri Kovács

OUTLINE OF THE PROBLEM

Severe traumatic head injuries produce various deficits that do not resolve completely. One of these pervasive cognitive deficits is slow information processing [1,2]. For the head-injured patient this means that many daily-life activities are performed with the feeling that he/she has not enough time to think and act properly. As a consequence, patients who have sustained traumatic brain lesions often complain that these activities become unpleasant and demanding [3]. From a more objective point of view, slow information processing after traumatic brain injury affects every stage of the information processing chain, so that in most cases it is appropriate to speak of 'general mental slowness' [2,4].

Because mental slowness has such wide-ranging effects it is a target for cognitive therapy. The purpose of this chapter is to provide the clinical practitioner with a framework for the training and the improvement of disabilities that are mainly a result of mental slowness.

In cognitive rehabilitation practice, until recently, 'process training' (Ponsford [5] uses the term 'directed stimulation'; van Zomeren and Fasotti [3] talk about 'stimulation therapy') was the training method of choice for cognitive impairments like slow information processing. Process training is based on the idea that cognitive deficits can be improved by direct stimulation of the brain structures involved in a particular cognitive process. For mental slowness, for example, exercises improving reaction times on several kinds of target stimuli presented on a video computer screen were seen as having a significant impact upon mental speed. The results of this type of training have repeatedly been called into question [6–8]. Three ideas underlying process training seem to be doubtful. The first is the idea that a psychological process or function can be improved by simply stimulating it (this is also called the 'mental muscle building' model of rehabilitation [9]). The second is the idea that the training results might generalize to several related skills in daily life. The last is the supposition that one can expect full restoration of function provided that process training is long enough and intense enough. Given the huge amount of process training programmes around the world, reports of their effectiveness have been negligible [10]. For this reason we have thought that it might be preferable to use another approach toward slow information processing. We have called this approach 'strategy training'.

In strategy training the aim is not to restore a lost process or function, but to teach a new compensatory strategy. The use of this strategy should allow the patient to compensate for his/her mental slowness and to minimize the disabilities and handicaps that mental slowness produces in everyday life. There are several essential differences between process and strategy training. Strategy training is above all aimed at compensating for disabilities caused by mental slowness, not at restoring normal cognitive speed [11]. Moreover, in process training repetitive drill-and-practice exercises, which resemble daily-life functioning only remotely, are often used, whereas in strategy training exercises are directly targeted at relevant problem behaviour. As process training is often implemented in an artificial environment (often through the use of microcomputers), generalization problems are quite frequent. The direct training of problem behaviour in strategy training reduces this problem.

The main idea behind strategy training for mental slowness is that the brain-injured patient must learn to regulate time pressure in several relevant situations in order to compensate for his/her mental slowness. This time regulation may be achieved through behavioural as well as more cognitive strategies. In the experimental studies that we are conducting at present, three different daily-life tasks affected by slow information processing have been chosen as a target for training: a verbal information intake task, preparing a meal and participation in traffic as a cyclist. In principle, strategy training should be applicable to every problem behaviour caused by slow information processing.

THEORETICAL MODEL

The specific framework of strategy training for slow information processing can be illustrated by analysing a complex cognitive task like traffic behaviour [12]. Traffic behaviour, like any other task, can be described as a hierarchically ordered set with three levels of subtasks differing in the amount of internal time pressure present (Table 11.1).

Table 11.1 Model of Michon [12], describing traffic behaviour in three hierarchically ordered levels

Strategic level	Decisions without any time pressure before task execution
Tactical level	Decisions with slight time pressure during task execution
Operational level	Decisions with much time pressure during task execution

The first level is called the strategic level. At this level, one is concerned with decisions that precede traffic participation (the choice of the route, for example). Because there is ample time to take these decisions, no internal time pressure is felt. The second level has been named the tactical level. At this level one tries to minimize traffic risks on the basis of one's own skills and one's own anticipation of impending traffic situations (riding slower in misty conditions, for example). Here, more time pressure is present because there is a clear time limit for the decisions one has to take. The third and final level is the operational level. This is the level at which one selects and executes actions from moment to moment in order to avoid concrete dangers in traffic. The probability of occurrence of late or inadequate reaction is high at this level, because several decisions have to be taken in a very short period of time. On the other hand, at tactical and strategic levels relatively few decisions have to be taken and time pressure is slight or even absent.

Following this line of reasoning, compensation for deficits at the operational level must take place at tactical and strategic levels. An example of this behaviour in traffic is when someone decides to avoid the rush-hour in order to filter in and overtake less frequently. The same logic can be applied to slow information processing in everyday life tasks. In strategy training, patients with traumatic brain injuries are taught to maximize decisions at tactical and strategic levels in order to avoid as many problems as possible at the operational level. The execution of complex cognitive tasks must be reorganized in such a way that time pressure is prevented as much as possible (strategic level). When this is not feasible by means of decisions at the strategic level only, patients can be taught to draw their own attention and that of the persons surrounding them to the impending information overload (tactical level) in order to compensate for time pressure.

Luria [13,14] has repeatedly claimed that attentional skills depend upon subvocal or internal language. Moreover, the above-mentioned complex cognitive reorganization involved in strategy training also presupposes a skilled use of internal language. We therefore used a shorter variant of self-instruction [15] as a training device in strategy training to trigger the use of the cognitive strategy. Three stages of the classic Meichenbaum procedure have been retained. In cognitive modelling the trainer demonstrates and explains aloud how the task should be performed. In the overt guidance stage the trainee instructs himself aloud while performing the task, the trainer only giving self-instructional cues when necessary. Finally, in the overt self-guidance stage the trainee performs the task and pronounces the self-instructional rules aloud.

In practice, implementing a compensatory strategy for mental slowness is more complex than simply teaching the brain-injured patient a set of self-instructional skills. In line with the ideas of Crosson *et al.* [16] we have also aimed strategy training at increasing the awareness of deficits in patient with closed head injury. The timing of the training stages was mainly derived from Ylvisaker *et al.* [11] and consists of three main stages (Table 11.2).

Table 11.2 Strategy training programme stages and their goals in increasing awareness of deficit [16]

Strategy training stages	Goal
1. Awareness of errors and deficits	Emphasis on increasing **intellectual** but also emergent awareness: letting a patient know there **is** a problem
2. Strategy acceptance and acquisition	Emphasis on increasing **emergent** but also anticipatory awareness: a patient has to recognize a problem and act accordingly
3. Strategy application and maintenance	Emphasis on increasing **anticipatory** but also emergent awareness: a patient has to foresee a problem in different but similar tasks

In a first stage, the main emphasis will be on the subject becoming aware of errors and deficits caused by slow information processing. Therapeutic measures are aimed at increasing intellectual and emergent awareness [16]. The goal in this stage is to teach the patient to discriminate between effective and ineffective performance. The patient is stimulated to become aware of his/her deficits and particularly of the implications of these deficits for task performance. Different means can be used to attain this goal. The patient may be asked to perform several training tasks without any help or coaching. This is followed by verbal feedback on what the patient does incorrectly and by explanation about where in the task time pressure is important. The trainer may also illustrate several examples in order to show that time pressure is an important aspect of task performance.

A second stage of strategy training concerns strategy acceptance and acquisition. This stage is aimed at convincing the patient that the strategy is helpful in accomplishing the task and at teaching the strategy. In this way emergent and anticipatory awareness are stimulated. To demonstrate the usefulness of the strategy the trainer can role play or show the errors that the patient makes on video. At this stage, the trainer may use examples such as lists, memos and tape recorders in order to show the patient that compensatory strategies are also widely used by people without head injury.

We have named the cognitive strategy which is taught in this second training phase Time Pressure Management (TPM). It basically consists of four rules which the patient has to learn by heart. If memory impairment impedes this, a prompt in the form of a file card with the TPM rules is shown to the patient. What follows are the main steps of TPM (Table 11.3).

Table 11.3 Time pressure management (TPM) as a cognitive strategy to compensate for mental slowness

Step 1	**Task analysis** and identification of time pressure
Step 2	**Planning** in order to prevent time pressure as much as possible
Step 3	**Emergency planning** to deal with information overload
Step 4	**Executing** the self-made plan

In the first step the patient has to ask him/herself if there is any time pressure in performing the task. For this purpose he/she has to identify the main actions of the task. Next, the patient has to ask him/herself which of the actions require rapid information processing, for example doing two things simultaneously in a short period of time.

In the second step the patient must ask him/herself which actions can be performed when time pressure is still slight. The patient must then instruct him/herself to pay more attention to the actions that have to be performed under time pressure. The third step consists of planning for the prevention of internal time pressure. This step consists of specifying and listing all the measures that the patient must take in case of impending information overload. The fourth and last step requires the patient to carry out the plan and pay particular attention to (1) the actions that must be performed under time pressure and (2) the emergency plan that he/she has to carry out in case of information overload.

The third and last stage of strategy training emphasizes strategy application and maintenance. It differs from the second stage in that training takes place under more distracting and difficult conditions. This is to ensure that the compensatory strategy is maintained in different circumstances. The aim of this stage is to practise the use of the strategy and to generalize it beyond the context of training. Besides emergent awareness, special emphasis is given to anticipatory awareness. In order to execute the task correctly extensive practice may be necessary. Once the strategy has been faultlessly applied, it should be used in several tasks of the same kind (e.g. preparing different types of meal). Using a variety of materials or activities requiring the same strategy under different conditions may be the next step.

Finally, the patient may be taught to cope with increased background noise, simulating real-life task conditions.

PRACTICAL AND THEORETICAL CONSIDERATIONS

It is obvious that compensatory strategies require substantial cognitive efforts and elaborate information processing. We believe this to be beyond the ability of many brain-injured patients. We have, therefore, introduced a number of medical as well as neuropsychological selection criteria in order to select mildly head-injured patients as candidates for strategy training with rather complex skills (like cooking or listening). The patients had to be between 18 and 50 years of age. The injury should have occurred at least 3 months previously and the duration of coma had to be at least 15 minutes. Patients with very severe neuropsychological disturbances such as amnesia, agnosia, apraxia or aphasia were excluded. Motivation and physical abilities had to be sufficient to join the programme.

Unfortunately, since the beginning of the strategy training in January 1992, the small numbers of eligible candidates and the particular difficulty forming homogeneous experimental and control groups have forced us to change the original design of the study. Formerly, our study on strategy training was planned as a randomized pre/post-test control-groups design. Actually only one of the tasks, the verbal information intake task, was conducted following this design. For the reasons just mentioned, the remaining tasks (cooking and traffic participation) were carried out following a single-case experimental design.

This modification of the experimental design has had some theoretical and practical implications which will be discussed in what follows. The first implication is that two kinds of strategy training are now being implemented. The more cognitively orientated training approach has already been outlined above. It depends heavily on the four cognitive steps that have to be remembered by the patient. The second training approach is related to the single-case experimental design and takes a more behavioural form. In other words, specific target behaviours are directly trained using behavioural modification techniques. The main difference between this kind of training and the cognitive approach is that a patient is not bothered with steps to remember every time he wants to perform a task. This has two advantages. Firstly, not too much strain is put on the limited information processing capacity and intellectual abilities of the head-injured patient. Secondly, the similarity between this approach and the one most people use naturally contributes to a relatively smooth learning process. Not many people use cognitive strategies consciously, because most of the time this is quite unnatural and very tiring.

A second implication in using two different experimental designs is closely related to the single-case design and the accompanying behavioural training approach. One could argue that the hope of generalization of training results is now lost, because no general strategy applicable to different tasks is used any more [18]. In this sense it is probably true that goals in rehabilitation have to be more modest than in the past. Rather than improving the cooking skills of a patient, for example, improving his/her monitoring behaviour during the preparation of a meal seems to be a more realistic training goal. It remains to be seen if this is the direction that rehabilitation will take in the near future [18,19].

A final implication of using two different experimental designs is concerned more with the viability of the study in a clinical setting [20,21]. For example, in the group study, pre- and post-study measures consist of:

- neuropsychological tests, especially those measuring mental speed (such as the Paced Auditory Serial Addition Task [22] and a visual choice Reaction Time task);
- psychosocial questionnaires about coping style, wellbeing and independency in daily activities (such as the Functional Activities Questionnaire [23]);
- behavioural observations of task performance in training conditions.

These measurements place a rather heavy burden on the normal clinical procedures and on the patient. The same can be said for the single-case design, where a patient has to be assessed every week. Very careful analysis of which outcome measures are relevant for the research hypotheses has to be balanced with considerations about assessment length and clinical acceptance. Moreover, problems related to the development of suitable behavioural measures, for such practical tasks as cooking, add to the difficulties of implementing such a strategy training in a rehabilitation setting.

TWO EXAMPLES OF STRATEGY TRAINING IMPLEMENTED IN OUR STUDY

Despite the above-mentioned problems in our study, training has been taking place since January 1992 using the two mentioned experimental designs. An example of the training of listening skills (the verbal information intake task) will now be given, in the hope that the reader can see how the presented model about traffic behaviour has influenced strategy training for slow information processing. In this training a patient sits in front of a video recorder and has to listen to a video-taped story, which will be repeated at least twice – at most four times. Before the patient starts to listen to the story he has to engage the attention of the therapist, who will use the four-step strategy. Together patient and therapist will articulate this strategy in relation to recalling the story and finally the patient is prompted to work out the strategy for himself, verbally explaining his/her moves. After this the patient starts to listen to the video-tape. Meanwhile the therapist watches carefully to see if the patient is using some steps of the strategy. Afterwards the patient is asked to reproduce as much information as possible, and this is scored. The therapist then discusses what went wrong in using the strategy. Our experience is that patients think they will remember the information, but when really put to the test reproduce very little (usually just 25% of the information the first time).

The TPM strategy outlined above and displayed in Table 11.3 consists of four concrete steps. The first step is asking yourself if you have to do more than two things at the same time in this task. If the answer is affirmative, the second step has to be taken. In this step a short plan is made beforehand, in which the patient works out what few simple steps he/she can perform to give him/herself more time to perform the task. One could, for example, decide to have a conversation with someone in a room where there is no background noise such as a radio playing, or one could ask one's conversation partner to speak at a slower rate.

A third and related step is a short outline of an emergency plan. This is the most important facet of the strategy: during conversation for example, the patient decides that he/she will interrupt the speaker as soon as he/she feels overwhelmed with information. It is explained to the patient that this feeling of overload must eventually be interpreted as an emergency signal which tells the patient to activate the emergency plan. One simple step in this emergency plan is to interrupt the speaker and ask for some reiteration or explanation. Another step would go further, requiring the patient to repeat the information.

The fourth and last step of TPM is simpler, but often forgotten by patients. It consists of actually executing the self-made plan and emergency plan. This last step seems rather trivial, but is far too often forgotten by patients. Such a dissociation between reasoning and doing is frequently demonstrated in closed-head-injury patients [13,14,24] and is probably due to a lack of insight or initiative [19,25]. In strategy training constant attention is paid to this failure of meta-cognition [11].

Several pilot studies with this kind of cognitive training indicate that even some of the most severely head-injured patients can eventually remember the four steps in the strategy, but some seem to find the execution of the plans extremely difficult. Cognitive impairments like lack of initiative or awareness, for a long time disregarded in the field of cognitive neuropsychology, seem to be playing a significant role in reported therapeutic successes [26].

The form TPM takes, in the above-mentioned strategy training, is a more active and assertive attitude towards a speaker during a listening task. Although this seems rather trivial, it still baffles us how little head-injured patients are aware of their passive attitude towards a complex task. They may have reached the stage of intellectual awareness [16], realizing that they cannot remember as well as they used to, but nevertheless when it comes to a simple listening task, they do not recognize their problem and take no preventive actions.

The training of preparing a meal (cooking) has quite a different form. Two kinds of target behaviours are trained sequentially in order to improve task performance. After intensive task analysis, we decided to train preparation and monitoring behaviour during the preparing of a meal. These two behaviours not only fitted in our strategy model [12], but were also identified by the occupational therapists as very important targets. Preparation consists of four steps, which can be taken to prevent time pressure during the cooking process as much as possible. For example, making a plan structures the task significantly (notice the resemblance with the cognitive training approach). Putting all ingredients and kitchen utensils on the table before one actually starts cooking diminishes for the most part the number of actions which have to be taken. Monitoring consists of certain control behaviours, like closely watching the time, checking the pans on the stove or the height of the flame. In a pilot study we have trained a patient using a single-case multiple baseline across behaviours ABCA-design. Figure 11.1 shows the results for the target behaviours 'preparation' and 'monitoring'.

Notice that the training only seems to have a positive effect on preparatory behaviour. This discrepancy may be explained by assuming that an improvement in preparatory behaviour reduces the need for monitoring behaviour. Moreover, preparatory steps are, for the most part, operant behaviours, whereas monitoring steps require higher-order cognitive processing. Presumably this last activity is more difficult for brain-injured patients. How improvement on these two target behaviours will eventually affect the quality of the meal still remains to be answered.

The training consists of working through some 15 standard recipes for one target behaviour and doing several simple assignments for the other target behaviour. Each target behaviour was trained for 3 hours! For example, in training preparation the patient is repeatedly asked to read a recipe very carefully and to write down all things which are needed in the cooking process. After this, setting up a global plan for task execution is

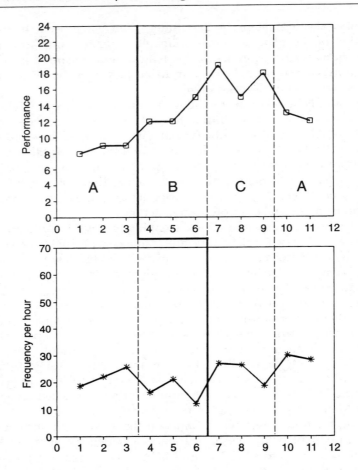

Figure 11.1 Single case multiple baseline across behaviours ABCA design for a head-injured patient. The thick line separates the baseline (A) from the training phase (B for 'preparatory behaviour', C for 'monitoring behaviour'). The top figure represents 'preparatory behaviour' and the bottom figure 'monitoring behaviour' during 9 weeks of 11 observations.

repeatedly practised. Examples are given by the occupational therapist and some situations are modelled. With the use of some behavioural techniques like shaping and positive reinforcement, a patient is stimulated to perform the necessary steps. The focus lies specifically on the target behaviour, which consists of some concrete behaviours, and in this way highly structured and repeated practice can be given. Monitoring is also trained with examples which are discussed extensively with the patient. For example, when the patient is performing an activity like cutting vegetables he/she has to check the pans on the stove regularly.

As Wood [27] has already pointed out, a behaviourally orientated training such as this has probably more to offer to a larger group of head-injured patients and is presumably applicable to a wider range of everyday tasks.

REFERENCES

1. Van Zomeren AH, Brouwer WH, Deelman BG. The riddles of selectivity, speed and alertness. In: Brooks DN, ed. *Closed Head Injury. Psychological, Social and Family Consequences.* Oxford: Oxford University Press, 1984.
2. Brouwer WH. Limitations of attention after closed head injury. Dissertation, State University Groningen, 1985.
3. van Zomeren AH, Fasotti L. Impairments of attention in brain-damaged patients. In: von Steinbuechel N, von Cramon DY, Poeppel E, eds. *Neuropsychological Rehabilitation.* Berlin: Springer Verlag, 1992.
4. Stocks LC, Gaillard WK. Task and driving performance of patients with a severe concussion of the brain. *Journal of Clinical and Experimental Psychology* 1986; **8**: 421–436.
5. Ponsford JL. Assessment and rehabilitation of attentional deficits following closed head injury. Unpublished PhD thesis, LaTrobe University, Melbourne, 1989.
6. Ponsford JL. The use of computers in the rehabilitation of attention disorders. In: Wood RL, Fussey I, eds. *Cognitive Rehabilitation in Perspective.* London: Taylor & Francis, 1990.
7. Ponsford JL, Kinsella G. Evaluation of a remedial programme for attentional deficits following closed-head injury. *Journal of Clinical and Experimental Neuropsychology* 1988; **10**: 693–708.
8. Robertson IH. Unilateral visual neglect. PhD thesis, University of London, 1988.
9. Harris JE, Sunderland A. A brief survey of the management of memory disorders in rehabilitation units in Britain. *International Rehabilitation Medicine* 1981; **3**: 206–209.
10. Wilson BA. Assessment and management of memory problems. In: von Steinbuechel N, von Cramon DY, Poeppel E, eds. *Neuropsychological Rehabilitation.* Berlin: Springer Verlag, 1992.
11. Ylvisaker M, Szekeres SF, Henry K et al. Topics in cognitive rehabilitation therapy. In: lvisaker MY, Gobble ER, eds. *Community Re-entry for Head Injured Adults.* Boston, MA: College Hill Press, 1987.
12. Michon JA. *Dealing with Danger.* Summary report of a workshop in the Traffic Research Centre, State University Groningen, 1979.
13. Luria AR. *Higher Cortical Functions in Man.* New York: Basic Books, 1966.
14. Luria AR. *The Working Brain. An Introduction to Neuropsychology.* New York: Basic Books, 1973.
15. Meichenbaum D. *Cognitive Behavior Modification. An Integrative Approach.* New York: Plenum Press, 1977.
16. Crosson B, Barco PP, Velozo CA et al. Awareness and compensation in postacute head injury rehabilitation. *Journal of Head Trauma Rehabilitation* 1989; **4**(3): 46–54.
17. Ylvisaker M. *Head Injury Rehabilitation: Children and Adolescents.* San Diego, CA: College-Hill Press, 1985.

18. Alderman N, Burgess PW. Integrating cognitive and behaviour: a pragmatic approach to brain injury rehabilitation. In: Wood RL, Fussey I, eds. *Cognitive Rehabilitation in Perspective*. London: Taylor & Francis, 1990.
19. Burgess PW, Alderman N. Rehabilitation of dyscontrol syndromes following frontal lobe damage: a cognitive neuropsychological approach. In: Wood RL, Fussey I, eds. *Cognitive Rehabilitation in Perspective*. London: Taylor & Francis, 1990.
20. Gonnella C. Designs for clinical research. *Physical Therapy* 1973; **53**: 1276–1283.
21. Wagenaar RC. Functional recovery after stroke. PhD Thesis, Free University Amsterdam, 1990.
22. Gronwall D, Wrightson P. Memory and information processing capacity after closed head injury. *Journal of Neurology, Neurosurgery, and Psychiatry* 1981; **44**(10): 889-895.
23. Pfeffer RI, Kurosaki TT, Chance JM *et al*. Use of the Mental Function Index in older adults: reliability, validity and measurement of change over time. *American Journal of Epidemiology* 1984; **120**: 922–935.
24. Goldstein K. The effects of brain damage on personality. *Psychiatry*, 1952; **15**: 245–260.
25. Lawson MJ, Rice DN. Effects of training in use of executive strategies on a verbal memory problem resulting from closed head injury. *Journal of Clinical and Experimental Neuropsychology* 1989; **11**: 842–854.
26. Prigatano GP. Disturbances of self-awareness of deficit after traumatic brain injury. In: Pritagano GP, Schacter DL, eds. *Awareness of Deficit after Brain Injury. Clinical and Theoretical Issues*. Oxford: Oxford University Press, 1991.
27. Wood RL. *Brain Injury Rehabilitation: A Neurobehavioural Approach*. London: Croom Helm, 1987.

Introduction to behavioural techniques for rehabilitation of brain-injured adults 12

Ann Goodman-Smith

INTRODUCTION

Behaviour disorders following severe brain injury can prevent rehabilitation. I first learnt this when I was working as a physiotherapist in a specialist neurological unit. It was there that I faced my first patient who had behaviour problems that prevented him from cooperating with physiotherapy. I became interested and remembered reading an article in *Physiotherapy* about the use of behaviour modification. I re-read it and decided to try and use the basic principles with the patient I was treating. His shouting and screaming behaviour was ignored by walking away, and positive reinforcement was given when he was quiet and cooperative. Having seen some encouraging results with this approach, I moved to work with the first of two teams I have been lucky enough to work with in specialized units. In both units, I have worked as part of a team, putting into practice behavioural programmes for severely brain-injured people [1]. So perhaps it is becoming clear that my background is one of a practitioner in the field of behaviour techniques with brain-injured adults. My background is not one of psychology with a detailed theoretical base to behavioural principles, but rather that of someone who has had experience of putting into practice those theories; this chapter is very much presented from that perspective.

It is important, however, to have some theoretical basis on which to hang the practical aspects of implementing behaviour techniques so, as Julie Andrews sings in *The Sound of Music*, 'Let's start at the very beginning ... with A, B, C.'

As behaviour is the subject under discussion, it is not difficult to guess that 'B' is behaviour. 'A' stands for antecedent – something that happens before a behaviour. 'C' is for consequence – what happens after the behaviour. 'A' – antecedent, 'B' – behaviour and 'C' – consequence.

'A' – ANTECEDENT

It is useful to look at the antecedents of a behaviour. For example, the antecedent to screaming behaviour might be that the person's arm was being passively stretched. Further investigation of this might show that the elbow had developed heterotopic ossification and that the procedure was causing pain. The subject of effective observation, accurate recording and measurement will occur later, but one cannot emphasize enough the importance of having as clear a picture as possible of the behaviour before starting to implement a behavioural programme. In this case of the antecedent being passive stretching of the joints, a behavioural programme might well not have been necessary because, having discovered the heterotopic ossification, a consequent change in the treatment would have occurred.

Another example is of a bus queue where people are patiently waiting – just as the bus approaches, a man runs up and jumps on to the bus, pushing others, who had been queuing patiently, out of the way. Clearly this behaviour is unacceptable to those in the queue. However, what they don't know is that the antecedent to this behaviour is the fact that the man has just heard that his wife has been rushed to hospital, having had a heart attack, and he is making his way as quickly as possible to join her at the hospital.

This, I think, demonstrates what may be the case in many instances; that there is nothing that can be done about the antecedent to the behaviour, but that it is the behaviour itself that will be the determining factor as to whether somebody is accepted in the community or not.

'B' – BEHAVIOUR

A wide range of behavioural disorders may occur as a result of severe brain injury. These can include verbal and physical aggression, non-cooperation, sexual disinhibition, lack of initiative and drive. The behaviour disorders may be as a direct result of injury to specific parts of the brain. For example, explosive temper outbursts may be due to damage to the temporal lobe and secondly they may be 'learned' behaviours so, for example, someone emerging from coma may start to call out. The natural reaction of the staff will be to respond to this by going to the individual to see what it is that is wanted. In behavioural terms, what happens by this response is that the calling-out behaviour is being rewarded by the attention that is being given to the individual by the staff. The result is likely to be that the shouting behaviour increases in frequency because it has been rewarded by the attention.

Some people will have behaviour disorders throughout the period of post-traumatic amnesia, but once an individual has emerged from this state the behaviour disorder does not persist. One of the first and important steps for the team to take is to recognize when a behaviour is impeding treatment. It is only after this recognition that the team can begin to do something about it.

It is all too easy to make excuses for the behaviour, but this will not necessarily be the swiftest course to the person's active participation in rehabilitation. Something must be done about it.

The 'B' in this ABC does not only mean behaviours that cause problems, such as those listed above, but it can also stand for behaviour in its broadest sense, which covers practically every function that we carry out. For example, one can think of walking behaviour, transferring behaviour, articulation behaviour. A behavioural approach can be successfully incorporated into specific therapies aimed at these behaviours and this approach creates a structured and effective way of re-learning these skills in rehabilitation [2].

'C' – CONSEQUENCE

A behavioural approach seeks to change behaviour, and the way that it does this is by looking at the consequence of the behaviour or what happens immediately after the behaviour occurs. If something rewarding happens immediately after the behaviour occurs, that behaviour is more likely to happen again. In order to increase the degree or frequency of the behaviour, positive reinforcement or a reward is given to increase the appropriate behaviour. To achieve this, the positive reinforcement needs to be given immediately and systematically in response to the desired behaviour. So, each time the behaviour happens, positive reinforcement needs to be given.

POSITIVE REINFORCEMENT

What is positive reinforcement? What is rewarding for the individual? My mind goes back again to *The Sound of Music* and Julie Andrews and another classic song, 'These are a few of my favourite things'. The behaviour will only increase if the reinforcement is rewarding to that individual.

It is therefore important to find out what are the things that he/she likes. So, for example, it could be inappropriate to play someone some pop music if their particular taste was in classical music or to give somebody Coca Cola or some other fizzy drink when they only like still drinks.

SOCIAL REINFORCEMENT

One of the most powerful reinforcers is social reinforcement. This is praise, a smile, a touch on the arm, attention. 'That was fantastic. You did that really well.' The delivery of this social reinforcement needs to be warm, enthusiastic, big and bold, particularly with this group of people who, because of their brain injury, may have reduced awareness and understanding. Over the years, with the teams I have worked with, one of our rules for delivering social reinforcement has been that it should be so big, bold and over the top it should make the person delivering it feel embarrassed.

OBLIQUE SOCIAL REINFORCEMENT

For some individuals it may be more appropriate to be less direct in delivery of social reinforcement, for those who don't respond well to a straight behavioural approach [3].

These are usually individuals who have suffered hypoxic or hypoglycaemic insults and whose behaviour is characterized by hysterical features. It appears they are almost driven to 'play games' and produce opposite effort. At Grafton Manor a less confronting approach has been developed, where the emphasis is on allowing appropriate behaviour to occur in a non-directive way and then giving oblique social reinforcement immediately after the behaviour occurs. An example of this is again giving attention, but the attention may be directed away from the task the person has just achieved. Instead it may be directed towards what the person is wearing, – 'That is a nice jumper you have got on today,' or 'Those are pretty earrings,' – or towards having a joke or, for an ardent football supporter, commenting that you saw his/her team win last night on the television.

TANGIBLE REINFORCEMENT

Tangible reinforcers are literally something that can be touched and are also sometimes called 'concrete reinforcers'. These can be things such as food, drink, tokens. A token is a small, round, plastic disk which is, in itself, not reinforcing! However, it is always given with social reinforcement and it is later exchanged for some sort of reward. Back-up reinforcers can be used in conjunction with social reinforcement, for example, at the end of a very good session aimed at improving posture and walking, a cool refreshing drink may be given.

An example of the use of tokens is that a half-hour period during rehabilitation can be divided into 2-minute intervals. At the end of the 2-minute period, if effort in the preceding 2 minutes has been achieved, a token is given. A baseline is first obtained before introducing tokens.

If the baseline shows that a tick was recorded in six out of the fifteen 2-minute intervals, a target of five ticks might be set so that if, at the end of the half hour, five tokens had been paid a reward would be given. If, however, four had been obtained, no reward would be given. The importance here is on setting the target at an achievable level, so that a reward can be given. Gradually the number of tokens needed to earn the reward is increased.

The reward at the end of the half-hour period can be whatever is rewarding and appropriate for the person and so, for example, it might be a drink, listening to a tape, having 5 minutes rest and a chat. Alternatively, a reward in this session might be linked into achievement throughout the sessions during the week, which might lead to a reward being given at the end of the week. For example, wallowing in a hot bath full of bath oils on Saturday morning, a lie in on Sunday with breakfast in bed and a Sunday newspaper, or a trip to the cinema on Saturday night.

TOKEN ECONOMY

In a token economy, tokens are given for acceptable behaviour. Most commonly this is on a time basis. For example, the day may be split into 15-minute periods or 30-minute periods and at the end of each of these periods the token is given with social reinforcement for the appropriate effort and behaviour.

Tokens are exchanged for various rewards; these might be drinks, leisure activities, free time. One of the advantages a token economy system does provide is an inbuilt structure which helps staff. The giving of a token at set intervals acts as a reminder to give the social reinforcement [4].

There is, then, a range of means of giving positive reinforcement. Each has its advantages and disadvantages, and the important thing is to use positive reinforcement, which is meaningful and appropriate for the individual and the programme.

So, positive reinforcement or a reward is given to increase the appropriate behaviour and the more often a behaviour occurs, the more opportunity there is to change it. The whole emphasis of a behavioural approach is that it is a rewarding system. The emphasis must always therefore be on the positive.

It is always important to remember this when using a behavioural approach, and it can be useful to have a way of illustrating the point – one that has been used before, is to quote the song, sung by Ella Fitzgerald, called 'Accentuate the positive'. If the consequence of the behaviour is rewarding, the behaviour is more likely to happen again, and each time the behaviour happens, positive reinforcement needs to be given immediately and systematically, in response to the desired behaviour.

The positive reinforcement also needs to be appropriate and meaningful to the individual. If the target behaviour was clear articulation, the first goal was to clearly articulate three words and the programme was to repeat this 30 times in a session, an appropriate and meaningful positive reinforcer might be a sip of a drink. Something less appropriate would be a sticky toffee that took more than 2 minutes to consume, as this would totally disrupt the remainder of the programme!

When using this powerful behavioural technique, it is important to plan what sort of positive reinforcement is going to be used and for a method to deliver it, which addresses the other key points that it should be contingent on the behaviour, appropriate, meaningful and consistently applied.

TIME OUT FROM POSITIVE REINFORCEMENT

Time out from positive reinforcement is used to decrease or extinguish the inappropriate behaviour. Time out from positive reinforcement means not rewarding the behaviour or totally ignoring the inappropriate behaviour. There are different way to achieve this. 'Time out on the spot' (abbreviated to TOOTS) may consist of ignoring an inappropriate behaviour or the person who is exhibiting the inappropriate behaviour. For example, if a person is asked to stand up and they respond with verbal abuse, the abuse is ignored and the instruction is repeated. Alternatively, when the person is asked to stand up and responds with verbal abuse, the person is ignored for a minute or two before the instruction is repeated.

Situational time out

An example of situational time out is where an individual may be removed from a group activity for a short period of time and then returned to it. For example, someone in a wheelchair who is disrupting a group by shouting and receiving positive reinforcement from other people in the group is wheeled outside the room for a few minutes and then returned to the group.

Time out room

A time out room is a small, non-stimulating room where an individual can be physically isolated for a short period of time to minimize the opportunity for positive reinforcement. Its most usual use is following an incident of physical aggression. This is because this is a behaviour that is difficult to ignore by the other methods described above. Although the use of the time out room is not designed for management, rather for treatment, there is no doubt that having a standard response to physical aggression acts as a great support for staff. It allows them to know how to respond in difficult, often frightening situations and must therefore have an effect on reducing their anxiety.

All the above are different ways of achieving time out from positive reinforcement in order to decrease or extinguish inappropriate behaviour. It is important to emphasize, however, that this will only work if it is used against a background of positive reinforcement. If the usual experience is not one of positive reinforcement, time out from positive reinforcement will not be a noticeable change. Removing a person from an unrewarding situation will not then have the effect of reducing the inappropriate behaviour.

Positive reinforcement and time out from positive reinforcement are the two main tools incorporated in a behavioural approach. The application of these two tools and the balance between them are crucial in the success of a behavioural approach.

Positive reinforcement and time out from positive reinforcement can only be introduced after other key features of a behavioural approach are put into practice.

OBSERVATION, MEASUREMENT AND RECORDING

OBSERVATION

Observation and accurate recording of behaviour and abilities enables change to be monitored in response to both the behavioural approach and to rehabilitation interventions. There are a number of ways of measuring and observing. Baseline information is of great importance. Baselines (which can mean writing down everything that a person does) may be geared towards specific activities, for example, a baseline of getting up, washed and dressed in the morning or a baseline of eating behaviour. Specific behaviours can, therefore, be highlighted and counted after interventions.

It is important to describe the behaviour accurately, so the rule is to describe what actually happened, rather than giving opinions. For example, it would be better to say 'He hit me on the arm,' rather than 'He became aggressive'. The first gives a much clearer description of what actually happened.

Similarly, an account of the number of times the behaviour happened is much more informative than words such as 'sometimes' or 'often'. 'He shouted four times today' is a much clearer description than 'He was often noisy'. Observation and measurement will help to define clearly the behaviours, which is an essential step in the planning process of introducing a behavioural programme. Indeed, one of the things that can go wrong in a behavioural programme is not defining clearly the target behaviour.

MEASUREMENT

One useful way of measuring and recording behaviour is a time sample. Rather than counting every time a behaviour happens, a sample of the behaviour is taken at different intervals throughout the day. This method is particularly appropriate for behaviours that occur frequently. The more frequently a behaviour occurs, the shorter the sample length can be. For a behaviour that is occurring very frequently, a 2-minute sample period might be appropriate, whereas, where the rate of the behaviour occurring is quite low, a sample of about 15–20 minutes might be necessary. The sample periods are spread out across the day and week so that representative information is gathered. A time sample may be used as a pretreatment baseline.

The programme may then be introduced and the time sample repeated a few weeks later. It would then be repeated in exactly the same way at the same intervals, and a comparison can then be made between the pretreatment baseline and the post-treatment sample. Depending on the behaviour being measured, it may be appropriate to record the duration of the behaviour. For example, if the behaviour was lying on the floor, in the sample period it might also be necessary to time how long the person was on the floor for.

For other behaviours, it would be sufficient simply to make a note at the time of the sampling with a tick or cross on the recording sheet, denoting whether the behaviour was occurring at that time. An example of where this might be used is where one is seeking to improve attention to a task. At each sampling, observation is made as to whether the person was attending to the task in hand.

A behaviour rating scale can be used to identify target or problem behaviours. At Grafton Manor, in order to emphasize the 'accentuate the positive' approach to using behavioural techniques, the behaviour rating scale has a positive side to it. The rating scale may be on a scale of 0–10, where 0 means the behaviour never occurs and 10 means it always occurs. A behaviour rating scale is used by a number of different members of the team. It is important to have a mix of people rating, as behaviours may be different with different people and in different situations.

For example, it is not uncommon that, when the patient is put under pressure to do physically difficult things in physiotherapy, physical aggression may occur, so the physiotherapist may well rate higher on this category than the speech and language therapist, who may not witness physical aggression during speech and language sessions. The scores from these scales can then be combined and expressed as a percentage. Behaviours can also be grouped under different headings, for example, aggression, sexual behaviour, motivation.

RECORDING

Accurately recording measurements is important if the information is to be useful. The simpler the recording methods, the more likely it is to be accurate. The design of recording sheets is very important. An example in Figure 12.1 shows a weekly points sheet, points being the social reinforcement in this case.

Here a code is used that relates to the patient's ability to earn. A daily total is scored, and then a weekly percentage obtained from the weekly total. The information is then transferred on to a graph, which gives a visual picture of progress. For recordings to be consistent and accurate, it is best to get into the habit of recording immediately. In Figure 12.2 a recording of a washing and dressing programme is shown.

The guidelines and recording sheet need to be clearly set out and any symbols being used should be clearly indicated; instructions for filling out the recording sheet need to be clear and concise.

SHAPING

Shaping is another behavioural technique. It means building desirable behaviour a step at a time. One of the important aspects of planning a behavioural programme is to give as many opportunities as possible for the behaviour to occur, so that there are many opportunities for giving positive reinforcement. The behaviour is going to increase in frequency because the consequence of the behaviour will be rewarding.

It is important to set the task at an achievable level, so that positive reinforcement can be given. It is often tempting to set the task higher, because one gets the feeling that the person can achieve at the higher level. However, it is most important that this does not happen with a behavioural approach, otherwise opportunities for giving positive reinforcement will be lost and the desired change in behaviour will not occur.

PROMPTING

Prompting can be used to initiate a behaviour. There are different sorts of prompts – physical, verbal and gestural. A physical prompt may consist of guiding a limb or part of the body, for example putting the

WEEK COMMENCING: _____   NAME: _____

REASONS FOR EARNING:

A. COMPLETING WASHING AND DRESSING WITHOUT HAVING TO DO AGAIN

B. COTTAGE BEING CLEAN AND TIDY

C. FEEDING POULTRY BEFORE DARK

D. PUTTING AWAY POULTRY BEFORE DARK

E. TAKING PILLS BY 10.00AM AND 8.00PM

F. ARRIVING AT SESSIONS ON TIME

G. PARTICIPATING IN SESSIONS

H. HAVING SPECTACLES WHEN PILL BOX IS CHECKED

Instructions:-

1. If points have been earned, place ✓ in relevant box

2. If any task from A - H not completed, place corresponding letter in box

TIME	MON	TUE	WED	THUR	FRI	SAT	SUN
8.00am - 9.00am							
9.00am - 10.00am							
10.00am -11.00am							
11.00am -12.00pm							
12.00pm -1.00pm							
1.00pm - 2.00pm							
2.00pm - 3.00pm							
3.00pm - 4.00pm							
4.00pm - 5.00pm							
5.00pm - 6.00pm							
6.00pm - 7.00pm							
7.00pm - 8.00pm							
8.00pm - 9.00pm							
TOTAL							

WEEKLY TOTAL _____   WEEKLY PERCENTAGE _____

Figure 12.1 A weekly points sheet.

NAME: WASHING AND DRESSING PROGRAMME

	MON	TUE	WED	THUR	FRI	SAT	SUN
TIME STARTED							
1. Get up							
2. Put on dressing gown							
3. Collect toiletries							
4. Go to the bathroom							
5. Turn on the taps							
6. Turn off the taps							
7. Get undressed							
8. Get into the bath							
9. Have a wash							
10. Wash your hair							
11. Get out of the bath							
12. Get dried							
13. Put on dressing gown							
14. Have shave/comb hair							
15. Brush your teeth							
16. Go back to your room							
17. Get dressed							
18. Make your bed							
19. Go downstairs							
TIME FINISHED							

GUIDELINES:

1. Give verbal prompt, as above,
   if necessary (maximum 3 prompts)

2. Give social reinforcement
   on completion of task

3. If no response on 3rd prompt,
   complete the task for him

RECORD:

✓   for social reinforcement
    given

P   for prompt

C   for task completed for him

Figure 12.2 Washing and dressing programme sheet.

foot to the opening of the shoe as a prompt to put the shoe on. Verbal prompts need to be concise and exactly the same each time. If the prompt was 'Put on your shoe', there should be no indication in the intonation of the voice that this is the 20th time this prompt has been repeated. It should sound exactly the same as the first time. It should not be a nag, as scolding and nagging can be rewarding and therefore positively reinforcing!

A gestural prompt may be used, and the same principles apply. An upward movement of the hand and arm may be used to indicate to the person to stand up, and a similar downward movement to indicate 'Sit down'.

Shaping and prompting can be illustrated in a programme aimed at increasing washing and dressing independence. Here the tasks involved are broken down into 20 stages. A prompt is given for each of the 20 stages and positive reinforcement, in the form of social reinforcement, is given for achievement for each of the tasks. Once the tasks start to be become established and achieved consistently, they can be grouped together, so the 20 tasks may become 14, then 8, then 3, until the entire process of getting up, washed and dressed and appearing at breakfast is achieved in one step. Obviously the phasing of this grouping, or 'chunking', needs to be gradual and done in such a way that the tasks or group of tasks are achievable, so that positive reinforcement can be given often.

MODELLING

Another way to help with initiation of behaviour is to model the behaviour. This happens often in life, in that we copy how others do things, so behaviour can be modelled and imitated and feedback given to the person. This is a technique that is often used in social skills training, which is an important part of the rehabilitation programme for many brain-injured people, whose social skills are impaired as a result of their injury.

At Grafton Manor, this technique is in operation frequently throughout the day. For example, at mealtimes team members will sit and eat at the same time and at the same tables as residents. In this way, appropriate social and eating behaviour is modelled.

So far, the behavioural techniques are fairly straightforward. However, as always, things aren't always as easy as they look!

SATIATION

Satiation is something to beware of. Overuse of a positive reinforcer has the effect of decreasing behaviour. One cannot go on giving the same positive reinforcer over long periods, unless it is still positively reinforcing. One of my colleagues demonstrated this admirably and bravely during a practical workshop, where the target behaviour was positively reinforced with the use of a rum truffle. The frequency of the desired behaviour started to increase, but after about the fifth rum truffle, satiation set in! This was a rapid and graphic representation of satiation, but often it is slower and creeps up on us, and so is something to watch out for on the recordings if the behaviour is decreasing instead of increasing.

CONSISTENCY

As you will have seen from the description of positive reinforcement, this needs to be given each time a behaviour occurs. Likewise, time out from positive reinforcement, to be effective, needs to be applied consistently.

In rehabilitation after severe brain injury, what this tells us is that, when using a behavioural approach, it is even more important to have a really good team working together, so that everybody knows which programmes are in operation, how to respond to specific behaviours and how to record them.

When setting up Grafton Manor, one of the things that was done was to look at all the potential barriers to a team working together. These include separate departments, titles which identify different disciplines, uniforms and hours of work [5].

Having identified these areas, the programme was planned to prevent the boundaries and emphasize the philosophy of sharing skills and blurring roles. All team members congregate in one room, where recordings and notes referring to each resident are kept. This is one way of working towards consistency by facilitating good communication. Programmes are only implemented following meetings, when many team members are present and have the opportunity to discuss and amend programmes. Regular formal and informal discussions happen, which helps to ensure everyone understands and agrees with individual programmes and can therefore apply them consistently.

Systems also need to be in operation to support the team and monitor the effectiveness of implementing the behavioural programmes, checking that 'accentuating the positive' is happening.

PLANNING AND IMPLEMENTING A BEHAVIOURAL PROGRAMME

A seven point programme is outlined below.

1. Assess and identify problem behaviour. The behaviour should be clearly and simply defined.
2. Measure it and record.
3. Plan contingent, positive reinforcement.
4. Plan contingent time out from positive reinforcement.
5. Implement programme.
6. Evaluate progress by repeating observation.
7. Alter reinforcement schedule as necessary.

This plan can be used as a guide when developing a behavioural programme, but emphasis should also be directed on accentuating the positive, setting realistic, achievable tasks and keeping the programme simple.

This chapter is an outline of the use of behavioural techniques in rehabilitation in brain-injured adults. It is aimed at being a guide to practising the use of these techniques, which can be effective in changing behaviour.

REFERENCES

1. Eames P, Wood R. Rehabilitation after severe brain injury: a special unit approach to behaviour disorders. *International Rehabilitation Medicine* 1985; 7(3): 130–133.
2. Goodman-Smith A, Turnbull J. A behavioural approach to the rehabilitation of severely brain-injured adults. *Physiotherapy* 1983; 69(11): 393–396.
3. Eames P. Hysteria following brain injury. *Journal of Neurology, Neurosurgery, and Psychiatry* 1992; 55: 1046–1053.
4. Turnbull J. Perils (hidden and not so hidden) for the token economy. *Journal of Head Trauma Rehabilitation* 1988; 3(3): 46–52.
5. Eames P, Turnbull J, Goodman-Smith A. Service delivery and assessment of programs. In: Lezak M, ed. *Assessment of the Behavioural Consequences of Head Trauma*. New York: Alan R Liss, 1989: pp 195–214.

He's no longer the same person:

how families adjust to personality change after head injury

13

Michael Oddy

INTRODUCTION

It is not only the families of head-injured people who have to adapt to sudden, long-term disability in one of their number. Spinal injuries, amputations and burns all occur suddenly in previously healthy individuals. Indeed many disabling illnesses may have a relatively sudden onset. However after head injury, although any or all functions may be affected, the most common and fundamental effects of head injury are to the higher functions. Changes in cognition and emotional responsiveness may alter the core characteristics of the person. Many studies have suggested that it is these changes in personality that cause relatives most distress. Rosenbaum and Najenson [1] compared the lives of wives of Israeli soldiers who had suffered a severe head injury with those of wives of soldiers who had suffered a spinal injury resulting in paraplegia. They found that the wives of head-injured soldiers were more disturbed by the changes than the wives of paraplegics. They disliked physical contact with their husband more than the wives of paraplegics and found their husband's disability more of a social handicap leading to a greater loss of contact with friends. Wives of the head-injured had significantly more symptoms of low mood. These findings have since been echoed by a number of studies [2–4]. Brooks and McKinlay [5] found that the influence of personality change on relatives' stress or 'burden' increased over time. Those relatives giving ratings of a high subjective burden were living with patients who were more quick tempered, unreasonable, mean, unkind, unhappy, apathetic, withdrawn and cold.

THE RANGE OF PERSONALITY CHANGES

One way of classifying these is to divide them into (1) those characterized by a loss of emotional control and (2) those that can be described as a loss of motivation. Kinsella *et al.* [6] found that among mothers of head-injured young adults emotional distress was closely related to their degree of loss of emotional control but not to loss of motivation. Weddell *et al.* [7] report a consistent finding that while the degree of friction in the family was not related to overall ratings of personality change it was related to the patients' irritability. Lezak [8], drawing on her extensive clinical experience, suggested five types of personality change most likely to create problems for families:

1. impaired social perceptiveness;
2. impaired control and self-regulation;
3. stimulus-bound behaviour;
4. emotional alterations;
5. inability to profit from experience.

Head injury covers a spectrum from the trivial to the fatal. Personality changes also occur in varying degrees and kind. Often such changes may be quite subtle and not immediately obvious, even to close friends or family who do not actually live with the head-injured person. Nevertheless, even subtle changes can make the person seem like a stranger, an imposter inhabiting the body of the person they knew.

There may be a **blunting of emotional feelings**. In certain respects this may appear a change for the better, in that the person may be more relaxed and less troubled by anxiety. They may be more easy-going, or unconcerned. On the other hand such people often experience less enjoyment or excitement and hence motivation to engage in activities they previously pursued with vigour may be lost. The effects on relatives may vary according to the nature of the relationship. However in the context of an intimate relationship this loss of feeling and concern may destroy the relationship.

Loss of inhibition is another common consequence of head injury. Once again it may occur in varying degrees. At the more subtle end of the spectrum it may involve a greater degree of outspokenness or a lack of judgement as to when certain jokes are appropriate. It is usually the relative who cringes with embarrassment, although the head-injured person may also realize their error, but only after the event.

A tendency to **inflexible concrete thinking** may make the person very difficult to live with. Such people tend to see issues in terms of black and white. They may become moralistic and develop strong opinions about quite trivial issues. They are intolerant of alternative opinions and where this is combined with memory deficits that prevent them from recalling previous discussions and agreements family life may become particularly trying.

Irritability and a tendency to lose one's temper more readily are among the most common personality changes after head injury. Perhaps because we all vary to some extent in these respects over time, these characteristics alone may be tolerated. However when they are in the context of other changes which have loosened the bonds of affection, it may be much harder for relatives to desist from responding in kind.

A number of changes in head-injured people mean that they have greater difficulty in maintaining social contacts. They may have difficulty in expressing themselves or at least doing so clearly and succinctly. They may have difficulty following conversations, attending to more than one person at once or picking up jokes. They may lose confidence and become withdrawn in social situations. The combined effect of these social handicaps is that they become more dependent upon their family for social support and contact [9]. The family are therefore often deeply involved in the care and support of their head-injured relative. However the person they are supporting and caring for is often perceived as a stranger. They have lost the person they loved, but gained responsibility for an unpredictable stranger. How do families adjust to such a strange situation?

THE PROCESS OF ADJUSTMENT

This process can be said to begin at the point the accident takes place, though it should not be forgotten that the length and nature of the previous relationship with the head-injured person will influence the process. It is during the immediate aftermath of the accident or injury that the family suffers the most acute distress. Within a few weeks, depending on the length of recovery, the distress subsides a little but remains at a high level indefinitely [3]. Indeed some studies have suggested that family distress increases as time goes by [10,11]. A more optimistic finding is reported by Novack et al. [12], who found that 33% of primary carers were clinically anxious and 9% clinically depressed at the time of admission of the head-injured person to the rehabilitation unit. By discharge this had reduced to 7% who were clinically anxious and 4% clinically depressed. A follow-up assessment 3 months later suggested that this improvement had been maintained.

In the early stages families may be fully aware only that the death of their relative is a possible outcome and the alternative is 'living'. This concept is not defined in any more detail than this. As the possibility of death recedes there is relief or happiness, with the automatic interpretation of survival as meaning full recovery. Although professionals are inclined to talk of denial this expectation of full recovery is not particularly surprising [13,14]. The families are unlikely to have encountered this situation before and thus have no knowledge upon which to base their expectations. Those involved in acute medical or surgical care tend to have only a hazy awareness of the likely outcome themselves. There is a natural tendency, even among professionals, to offer reassurance rather than accuracy. Certainly relatives will tend to listen more to what they wish, desperately, to hear. It may be only months, even years, later that they remember and understand more cautious information. One mother was told, 'In some ways it would be better if these head-injured people died, then you could grieve in public'. At the time she thought this a terrible thing to say. Now, 3 years later, she understands exactly what was meant. 'Now I grieve every day.'

As time goes by and the relative still hopes for a full recovery, a failure to return to normal is often interpreted as lack of cooperation [15]. Polinko et al. [16] suggest that during this stage what is required from professionals is empathic listening, repetition and structuring of information and reassurance. In the early stages of recovery the relatives will be struggling to form a clear picture of what their drastically altered future holds. Family members may need to be given 'permission' to express their hopes and fears for the future [17]. It is important not to bombard the family with information, but they will undoubtedly be asking questions. Frequently their understanding of the information they have been given will differ from that of the information-giver. Relatives will experience and express inconsistent views. It is important for the professional to see this as a process in which it takes time for a clear picture of the future to emerge. Certainly the information it is possible to give will change over time as the patient's eventual outcome becomes easier to predict.

The relatives may be able to appraise the situation differently by being encouraged to see specific symptoms or problems in a different light. For example, the extent to which the head-injured person has control over various aspects of his/her behaviour is frequently an important issue to address. If the relative sees the head-injured person's frequent memory lapses as being deliberately awkward or unhelpful they are likely to be irritated and react with anger. On the other hand if they view the person as being unable to remember anything, they may be unduly cautious and overprotective and inhibit the person's progress. Usually it is important to help relatives towards a balanced view whereby the head-injured person is seen as having major difficulties in certain areas, but still having some residual capability, the extent of which will vary from case to case.

In the later stages, relatives begin to realize that the person will not return to their previous state. As recovery tails off the relative is often able to develop a clearer picture of the nature of the changes. Anticipation of the future becomes easier, if more daunting. The recognition of personality changes appears to increase over time [5], presumably as a consequence of observing the head-injured person in a wider range of situations.

COPING WITH STRESS

There is a widely accepted view that certain families 'cope' better with the stress of caring for the head-injured person than others. Before proceeding further with this question it is important to briefly consider what it meant by the notion of 'coping'.

One potentially fruitful avenue of research has been to try to identify those factors that enable some to cope while others fail to do so. However the concept of coping is problematic. What do we mean when we say someone is coping? Do we mean the patient is thriving and being cared for appropriately? This is clearly a laudable aim, but is it the sole criterion irrespective of the costs to the relative or family? Does coping imply that the carer is maintaining his/her own health or emotional wellbeing? Do we consider that a carer is coping unless or until he/she becomes physically ill or has a nervous breakdown? Do we consider carers coping unless or until they simply refuse to carry on or decide to leave? It is probably true to say that families are often assumed to be coping if they are not making demands on external services.

The term 'coping' may refer to the relative having adjusted psychologically or emotionally to the changes in the head-injured person, and hence in their family life. Such adaptation perhaps more usually takes the form of resignation rather than acceptance. In practice it is likely that in the long term a person will only be able to cope in a stressful situation if two conditions are met. First, at least some of his/her personal needs must be met. Second, his/her aspirations must be broadly in line with what is possible, if only for short-term goals.

COPING AS A PROCESS

As well as asking 'Are you coping?' we frequently ask 'How are you coping?' Although it has not always been made explicit, most of the research in this area has been directed towards discovering what strategies relatives adopt to cope with the enforced changes in their lives. The aim has been to identify strategies that are successful and can be passed on to other relatives who may be currently employing less successful methods [18].

One major problem with this approach is the need to devise a means of classifying strategies by extracting essential features and to avoid simply generating an endless list.

The most commonly used classification is that proposed by Folkman and Lazarus [19]. This divides strategies into 'emotion-focused' and 'problem-focused'. The latter involve practical, problem-solving attempts and it appears that such strategies tend to be employed where change is perceived as a possibility. Emotion-focused strategies involve alterations to the way a problem is viewed or a direct attempt to alter the emotional response. Such strategies tend to be employed where the individual perceives the situation to be unalterable.

Examples of these types of response can be seen in the families of the head-injured.

Common 'problem-focused' strategies include generating home-based rehabilitation programmes, perhaps based on behaviour modification techniques described in the preceding chapter, where the relative helps the head-injured person through a series of often vigorous and usually physical exercises. It may also involve family members taking on a case management function or becoming deeply involved in setting up or supporting voluntary organizations dedicated to helping the head-injured.

'Emotion-focused' strategies often involve finding a way to restrict or alter the way the situation is perceived. For example one mother said she never thinks of her daughter as she was before the accident as this is too painful. Instead she concentrates on her daughter as she now is and tries to avoid seeing any links between the current and the former. In contrast to this mother, some relatives stress the aspects of the head-injured person that remain the same as before. The extent to which relatives emphasize the continuities or discontinuities in the person's personality is likely to have a major bearing on the way they cope.

Professionals have a tendency to criticize families as either being 'overprotective' or 'denying' the problems. In fact these two characteristics can be seen as opposite ends of the same dimension. Overprotection occurs as a result of the relatives overemphasizing the patient's disability. Denial results from the underemphasis of any disability. In terms of the coping mechanisms described above, overprotection can be seen as a problem-solving strategy while denial is an emotion-focused strategy. Professionals should however beware of jumping to conclusions of this kind. Certainly there are cases where the degree of overproduction is both unnecessary and inhibits progress. Similarly, there are occasions when denial of disability means that no attempt is made to overcome it. Caution is necessary because the family is invariably in the best position to observe the patient's capabilities and to judge the best balance between the need for hope and reality on the part of both themselves and the patient.

Personality changes may be extreme and complete or they may be subtle and partial. The relative's perception of the extent of this change may vary not only according to the 'objective' nature of the changes but depending upon whether they tend to focus on those aspects of the person that have changed or those aspects that remain familiar. This in turn may of course depend partly on the nature of the changes. For example where a kind, placid person has become violent and abusive, this aspect of their behaviour may eclipse other aspects which may have undergone less change. On the other hand if those aspects of the person's previous personality for which the relative had most affection are still present, the impression of the extent of change may be less. It is common for relatives of severely head-injured people to express the view that the person they previously knew and loved is simply no longer present. Instead a stranger with far less likeable characteristics inhabits their body. The relative is therefore in the position of not only having to grieve the loss of the person they loved, but also having to learn to live with a stranger. Spouses, while still grieving the loss of the original partner, are expected to embark on an intimate sexual relationship with a stranger who has replaced the partner. The head-injured person him/herself often feels that little has changed and finds it very hard to understand the reluctance of the spouse. The issue of their sexual relationship frequently becomes a focus of tension and argument. Such relatives will commonly say that they would willingly fulfil the role of carer but cannot continue in the role of sexual partner. This results in a 'head-on' conflict which not infrequently results in sexual violence, even when aggression is not a major problem outside the sexual relationship.

For all the relatives of head-injured people who have suffered a significant personality change, the question arises as to whether they can continue to live with the head-injured person. Many do stay together simply because neither they nor the head-injured person have anywhere else to go. This is perhaps particularly so for parents of head-injured people, since for them there is no equivalent of divorce or separation. Among married head-injured people divorce rates are indeed high. Tate *et al.* [20] found that 6 years after head injury 17 out of 31 couples had divorced. It seems that, where people have children, the rate is far higher. Thomsen [21], in a 15-year follow-up, found that of nine couples, only two remained married. Both of these couples were childless, whereas all of those who had parted had children. It may be that the presence of children helped to resolve the dilemma for the uninjured spouse. When the decision is based on the balance of benefit to themselves or to their head-injured partner, they may find it impossible to take the decision to put their own interests first. However when the interests of children are weighed in the balance the arguments for separating may be heavier. There is also more likely to be support and understanding from other members of the family and friends if the decision is made on the basis of the wellbeing of children.

THE MAJOR ISSUES FACING FAMILIES

One particular relative, the partner of a head-injured man, came to a consultation with the author armed with a list of clearly stated questions. These questions encapsulate the dilemmas faced by most relatives although they are rarely so clearly and comprehensively stated.

- Am I personally capable of taking on this life of caring for David? Can I do it?
- Are there techniques I can learn that will help me to cope?
- Have I exhausted the support that might be available from other agencies?
- If I do not have him back, what will happen to him?
- If I do decide not to have him back, how will I get him to understand and accept my decision?
- How important am I to him? Will he make more progress or be happier and better able to adjust to his disabilities if I am there to help him?

It should be stated that in the present author's view there are no right or wrong answers to these questions. However the professional advisor, with a knowledge of head injury and its effects on family life, may be able to play a valuable role in helping relatives who are 'stuck' in their deliberations. Relatives commonly find very little opportunity to discuss these issues with an informed and understanding other. Close friends will have little appreciation of the experience of living with a brain-injured person and may particularly fail to appreciate the difficulties if the person seems perfectly well recovered on superficial contact. The same is true for close relatives not actually living in the home. And here there is the added difficulty of their emotional involvement and distress, which frequently leads to disagreement and bitterness between different factions of the close family. This is especially common between spouses and the patient's parents.

AM I PERSONALLY CAPABLE OF TAKING ON
THIS LIFE OF CARING?

The question 'Will I be able to cope?' cannot be answered directly. However there are certain factors which clearly make the situation more difficult. A careful examination of these may help the relative to reach a more rational decision. For example, the study cited earlier suggests that the presence of children is an important consideration. Their interests will need to be given top priority. While studies have failed to show any major differences between spouses and parents or other relatives [3,10,22], spouses clearly need to decide whether they feel able to continue a sexual relationship with their injured partner. If they do not feel able to do so immediately a great deal of work will often be necessary to help the patient understand this, or at least to arrange matters in a practical way in order to minimize the potential friction.

The length and quality of the relationship prior to the injury is also likely to influence the ability to cope with a care-giving role, though not perhaps as much as the amount of affection felt for the injured spouse [23–25]. The amount of social support available from friends and extended family should also be considered. Financial circumstances, quality of housing and other stresses in the family will also have a bearing. Will it be possible for the uninjured relatives to continue to work or will they have to give up this aspect of their lives to care for the injured member? The specific presentation of the head-injured person also requires consideration. Does he or she have uncontrolled verbal or physical outbursts? Is his/her behaviour repetitive in a wearing way? Is he or she very rigid and difficult to reason with? What redeeming features does he or she possess? How has the uninjured relative responded to stressful circumstances in the past?

ARE THERE TECHNIQUES I CAN LEARN TO HELP ME COPE?

Once of the most influential theories of coping is that developed by Lazarus and colleagues [26]. This postulates a two-stage process. In the first stage of primary appraisal the person makes a judgement as to whether the situation or circumstance he or she encounters is relevant to his/her wellbeing. If it is, is it benign or stressful? Stressful events include, threats, challenges or actual harm or loss. If the situation is seen as stressful, appraisal takes place at a secondary level and the person assesses his/her coping resources. This model suggests two major strategies for helping relatives to cope. One involves altering the way they appraise the situation and the other enhancing their ability to deal with it. Altering their appraisal of the situation involves the provision of information, either directly or through a counselling process. The nature of this information will vary according to the stage after injury. Enhancing the relatives' ability to cope with the situation includes direct attempts to reduce the problem through the rehabilitation of the patient. However it also includes training relatives in methods of management or rehabilitation.

There are a wide variety of ways in which relatives may continue or consolidate the work of rehabilitation personnel. The use of regular structured routines that depend upon the normally less impaired procedural memory is important. Behaviour modification techniques to limit behavioural problems may be appropriate. These involve techniques to avoid eliciting the behaviour as well as methods of responding when inappropriate behaviour occurs and are discussed in more detail in

Chapter 12. It is often helpful to encourage relatives to see all their efforts as experimental and to encourage them to define desired outcomes and collect information in order to assess changes [27]. Helping relatives to understand the often altered needs of the patient may enable them to meet these appropriately. Previously very energetic individuals may after head injury be quite content to lead much more restricted and apparently monotonous lives. They may find social or other activities a great strain and relatives may need to be dissuaded from pushing too hard to ensure they lead full and active lives.

HAVE I EXHAUSTED THE SUPPORT THAT MIGHT BE AVAILABLE FROM OTHER AGENCIES?

In an area where services are extremely patchy if not entirely absent there is a clear need for relatives to be made aware of those services that do exist, both dedicated head-injury services and appropriate services for other or wider client groups (Chapters 4 and 5). The type of support available will include financial and practical support, social and emotional support and specialized professional support.

All professions involved with the head-injured have a responsibility to ensure that relatives are directed to the appropriate people and places to ensure that this advice is forthcoming. The advent of the case manager [28] should facilitate this process. However, the professional advisor will on occasions have to tell the family that there may be little to be gained by seeking advice from further agencies. Understandably, families will tend to look hopefully towards more and more experts in an attempt to find answers that may not exist.

HOW IMPORTANT AM I TO HIM?

There are two aspects to this question. One concerns the issue of the nature of the personal relationship. The other concerns the extent to which the family can affect the process of recovery. The latter is potentially an empirical question, which could be answered by research. Unfortunately, there is little research that addresses this issue, although many writers have emphasized the importance of the family in the rehabilitation process. It is likely that the family can be influential in encouraging and motivating the patient in his rehabilitation efforts. Where such efforts are a sufficient condition for success the family's role in this respect is of paramount importance. However, more often motivation alone is not sufficient and will result in relatively minor gains. In these situations Lezak [8] has stressed that it is important to emphasize to family members that there is relatively little they can do to influence the patient's recovery.

The relative is likely to have experienced a profound change in the nature of their personal relationship with the head-injured person. It seems clear that the head-injured person too often experiences such a change. Despite this, head-injured people normally cling tenaciously to their family relationships. In the presence of severe memory deficits and concrete and perseverative thought processes it is extremely difficult to know exactly what impact separation from members of the family has on the head-injured individual.

IF I DO NOT HAVE HIM BACK WHAT WILL HAPPEN TO HIM?

This question again can be answered both in terms of the patient's emotional response, their general progress and more practically in terms of where they will live, how they will cope on a day-to-day basis. A knowledge of available local services may enable the professional to advise relatives in this respect and help them to develop a more detailed picture of what such a future would mean.

IF I DECIDE NOT TO HAVE HIM BACK HOW WILL I GET HIM TO UNDERSTAND AND ACCEPT MY DECISION?

Any discussion of this issue will clearly depend on the nature of the head-injured person's deficits. In many cases it may be necessary to advise the relative that it is unlikely to be possible to help the injured person to understand and accept the decision. This question may reflect the ambivalence, the feelings of responsibility and guilt on the part of the relative. The best way of tackling such a question may be to discuss it in these terms.

CONCLUSIONS

Families of those suffering personality changes as a result of their head injuries, even where these changes are subtle ones, face alarming decisions and major obstacles in forging a satisfactory new life for themselves and the patient. Frequently they are forced to do this alone as few will appreciate the nature of the emotional and practical problems they face. The opportunity to meet others who are having or have had similar difficulties is for some the most helpful approach. Ideally all professionals dealing with head injury should have some awareness of the circumstances relatives confront. This would help avoid misunderstandings and misinterpretations and assist in the joint search for solutions to practical problems. The availability of an aware professional may also be of considerable value when, as is often the case, family and friends are not able to fulfil this role.

REFERENCES

1. Rosenbaum M, Najenson T. Changes in life patterns and symptoms of low mood as reported by wives of severely brain-injured soldiers. *Journal of Consulting and Clinical Psychology* 1976; **44**: 881–888.
2. Thomsen IV. The patient with severe head injury and his family. A follow-up study of 50 patients. *Scandinavian Journal of Rehabilitation Medicine* 1974; **6**: 180–183.
3. Oddy M, Humphrey M, Uttley D. Stresses upon the relatives of head-injured patients. *British Journal of Psychiatry* 1978; **133**: 507–513.
4. Florian V, Katz S, Laman V. Impact of traumatic brain damage on family dynamics and functioning: a review. *Brain Injury* 1989; **3**: 219–233.
5. Brooks DN, McKinley WW. Personality and behaviourial change after severe blunt head injury – a relative's view. *Journal of Neurology, Neurosurgery, and Psychiatry* 1983; **46**: 336–344.
6. Kinsella G, Packer S, Olver J. Maternal reporting of behaviour following very severe blunt head injury. *Journal of Neurology, Neurosurgery, and Psychiatry* 1991; **54**: 422–426.
7. Weddell R, Oddy M, Jenkins D. Social adjustment after rehabilitation: a two year follow-up of patients with severe head injury. *Psychological Medicine*, 1980; **10**: 257–263.
8. Lezak M. Living with the characterologically altered brain injured patient. *Journal of Clinical Psychiatry* 1978; **39**: 592–598.
9. Kinsella G, Ford B, Moran C. Survival of social relationships following head injury. *International Disability Studies* 1989; **11**: 9–14.
10. Livingston M G, Brooks DN, Bond MR. Patient outcome in the year following severe head injury and relatives' psychiatric and social functioning. *Journal of Neurology, Neurosurgery, and Psychiatry* 1985; **48**: 876–881.
11. Brooks DN, Campsie L, Symington C *et al*. The 5 year outcome of severe blunt head injury: a relative's view. *Journal of Neurology Neurosurgery, and Psychiatry* 1986; **49**: 764–770.
12. Novack TA, Bergquist TF, Bennett G *et al*. Primary caregiver distress following severe head injury. *Journal of Head Trauma Rehabilitation* 1991; **6**(4): 69–77.
13. Romano M. (1974). Family response to traumatic head injury. *Scandinavian Journal of Rehabilitation Medicine* 1974; **6**: 1–4.
14. Novack TA, Richards JS. Coping with denial among family members. *Archives of Physical Medicine and Rehabilitation* 1991; **72**: 521.
15. Lezak MD. Psychological implications of traumatic brain damage for the patient's family. *Rehabilitation Psychology* 1986; **30**: 241–250.
16. Polinko P, Barin J, Leger D *et al*. Working with the family. In: Ylvisaker M, ed. *Head Injury Rehabilitation: Children and Adults*. Boston, MA: Little, Brown, 1985: pp 93–115.
17. Rosenthal M, Young T. Effective family intervention after traumatic brain injury; theory and practice. *Journal of Head Trauma Rehabilitation*, 1988; **4**: 42–50.
18. Suls J, Fetcher B. The relative efficacy of avoidant and non-avoidant coping stategies: a meta-analysis. *Health Psychology*, 1985; **4**: 249–288.
19. Folkman S, Lazarus RS, Dunkel-Schetter C *et al*. Dynamics of a stressful encounter; cognitive appraisal, coping and encounter outcomes. *Journal of Personality and Social Psychology* 1986; **50**: 992–1003.

20. Tate R, Lulham JM, Broe GA *et al*. Psychosocial outcome for the survivors of severe blunt head injury. *Journal of Neurology, Neurosurgery, and Psychiatry* 1989; **52**: 1128–1134.
21. Thomsen IV. Late outcome of very severe blunt head trauma; 10–15 year second follow up. *Journal of Neurology, Neurosurgery, and Psychiatry* 1984; **47**: 260–268.
22. Brooks N, Campsie L, Symington C *et al*. The effects of severe head injury upon patient and relative within seven years of injury. *Journal of Head Trauma Rehabilitation* 1987; **2**: 1–13.
23. Zarit SH, Todd PA, Zarit JM. Subjective burden of husbands and wives as caregivers: a longitudinal study. *Gerontologist* 1986; **26**: 260–266.
24. Lezak M. Brain damage is a family affair. *Journal of Clinical and Experimental Neuropsychology* 1987; **10**: 111–123.
25. Morris RG, Morris LW, Britton PG. Factors affecting the emotional wellbeing of the caregivers of dementia sufferers. *British Journal of Psychiatry* 1988; **153**: 147–156.
26. Folkman S, Lazarus RS. An analysis of coping in a middle aged community sample. *Journal of Health and Social Behaviour* 1980; **21**: 219–239.
27. Zarit SH, Zarit JM. Families under stress; interventions for care givers of senile dementia patients. *Psychotherapy; Theory, Research and Practice* 1982; **19**: 461–471.
28. McMillan TM, Greenwood RJ, Morris JR *et al*. An introduction to the concept of head injury case management with respect to the need for service provision. *Clinical Rehabilitation* 1988; **2**: 319–322.

Making group work work

14

Debora Prichard and Eric Bérard

BACKGROUND

Our personal experience in brain injury rehabilitation has led us to create various rehabilitation–readaptation approaches with groups of patients, with the aim of helping them and their families find a psychosocial adjustment to their new and often difficult situation [1–8].

Indeed, on the one hand, personality and emotional disturbances, often encountered after traumatic brain injury, contribute greatly to the family burden [9]; on the other hand, the image the brain-injured person has of his mind and body must be adjusted to fit the new situation. Analogies may be drawn with the development of the child, who has to adapt his own body image to his changing body [10], as well as the teenager's development when he has to discover his identity with respect to others in order to move from narcissistic behaviour to an objective relationship. In the same way, traumatic brain-injured patients have to re-establish their own identity [4]. Furthermore, their new behaviour may be often characterized by regression, which hinders communication and relationship with others and which hinders their reacceptance into the community.

Taking into account the psychosocial adjustments that must be made, we have proposed two different approaches, both using the dynamics created from a group situation. Our earliest attempts were inspired by certain psychodrama techniques. We know from psychodrama that anyone 'playing a role' may feel able to express something he/she would not communicate under normal circumstances [1]. One of our experiences in leading a group of TBI patients, playing various roles behind a mask, led us to discover the importance of being able to 'run away from reality'. But we also realized that there was a genuine desire among the TBI patients to face real situations such as the possibility of returning home. The first experience of returning home often ends in failure, because patients have to adjust both to their new identity and to the reactions from their unprepared relatives, who often have great difficulty accepting the changes incurred from the accident [3]. Psychodrama and other types of group dynamics can help patients, by interacting with others, to adjust to their new identity as well as to the reactions from those around them [3,7].

A second approach is inspired from drama–theatre techniques, coupled with the teaching possibilities of using 'active' learning [6,8]. The ultimate aim of this approach is also to help the brain-injured patient readjust to his new image and the reactions of others. This approach is more pragmatic in nature than the previous one; we try to set specific, measurable goals for each group of patients. We are currently exploring the various possibilities offered by this approach, and our account of the development of these techniques is the main core of this chapter.

Neuropsychological tests and theoretical models of rehabilitation can give therapists ways of creating specific rehabilitation exercises, but they are usually not ways of preparing patients, on a practical level, for returning into the community. Group work is a way of complementing other rehabilitation techniques. Being a competent group facilitator is difficult and requires both appropriate training and sufficient experience. That is the reason why we propose this practical demonstration of 'how to make group work work'.

PRACTICAL GUIDELINES FOR SUCCESSFUL GROUP WORK

PRELIMINARIES: SETTING UP YOUR GROUP

Before outlining some general group dynamic techniques, certain basic questions concerning the future group must first be answered. After analysing the reasons for proposing group work, the organizational aspects of the programme will be considered: choosing the participants, deciding on the frequency and duration of the sessions as well as where they will take place, setting objectives and subsequent programme contents. These points should, of course, be taken into account before any rehabilitation work (or any teaching for that matter), but it is an obvious step which is often overlooked. It would seem all the more important to consider these questions carefully when deciding to do group work with brain-damaged individuals. The answers to these questions may vary widely, but we shall try to provide a general framework, followed by specific examples gleaned from our personal experience.

Justification

Why should one do group work? Many medical directors or managers would, undoubtedly, like to know that group work is more economical than individual therapy, calculating that time and money can be saved if one or two therapists work with six to eight patients at the same time. However, it is essential to insist on the fact that the type of group work proposed in this chapter is qualitatively different from individual work. It is not putting eight individuals together and having them all do the same thing; that would simply be individual work done collectively. Group work is a complement to individual therapy, but by no means replaces it. Certain objectives may be the same, but the means of achieving them are always different.

If group work cannot replace individual therapy, what are its aims? The aim of most group dynamic techniques is to help the individual become aware of his potential. This kind of work, which can be beneficial for any individual, is crucial for the brain-damaged person, who must come to terms with his new 'self'. He must realize and accept his limitations, but even more importantly must discover his resources. In individual therapy, each therapist can help the patient discover his limits and capabilities within himself, but not as a part of a social structure, interacting with others.

Group work can therefore:

- create specific 'social environments', which can help each patient come to terms with his changed-but-somehow-the-same self; it can help the patient accept new limits, but also discover unsuspected resources;
- help the patient find his 'role' and 'place' in a controlled social setting; he can discover that he is not only a 'receiver' but can also be a 'giver', re-establishing alternating roles in a communication exchange;
- be a stepping stone on the road to establishing the patient's autonomy, an intermediate step between the privileged, protected and secure one-to-one relationship the patient has with his various therapists and the uncertainties and unknowns of the outside world he will have to face upon discharge.

Group work lends itself to richer, more fulfilling activities: the activities proposed come closer to obeying normal communication strategies as opposed to the repetitive and often artificial exercises usually done during individual therapy. Wonder of wonders, rehabilitation can even be enjoyable!

Choosing the participants

For which patients is group work most beneficial? Generally speaking, group work is best suited to patients ready to come to terms with their 'social self', manifesting a desire to communicate with others. Before beginning a group, each future participant is contacted individually. The objectives of the group programme are clearly presented and the patient decides at this point whether or not to participate.

The more homogenous the group, in terms of the impairment to be treated, the easier it is to define the objectives for group work. For the cohesion of the group, it is best if the same participants start and end the cycle together; it is difficult to add new members once the cycle has begun unless the group meets over a relatively long period of time.

Our experience has shown us that the choice of patients can vary widely, depending on the objectives of the group. We have, in fact, done group work at all stages of recovery.

- At an extremely early stage, we have organized groups dubbed 'stimulation groups'. It is not really pertinent to talk about group dynamics and social interaction *per se*, but this type of 'group' can be considered a preliminary stage. The participants are patients who have regained consciousness after a prolonged coma and are just beginning to establish a communication code, often paraverbal. It is the beginning of the awareness that others exist, and each participant, by his/her mere presence, is part of the group.
- Another group, which can be created at a relatively early stage, is one where the main objective is to develop each member's attention and concentration span, focusing on listening and paying attention to specific stimuli as well as to the other members of the group.
- When patients will soon be discharged, we organize groups that are aimed at being a springboard to help them take the last steps towards the autonomy necessary for independent living. These groups usually aim at developing decision-making and logical planning strategies, as well as action plans to implement their decisions.

Linked to the question of the choice of participants is the question of the number of members in a group. It is generally accepted that, for a maximum amount of group interaction and dynamics, a group should have between eight and 12 participants. Our experience has shown us that, with traumatically brain-injured adults, the optimal number is between six and eight, although we have reduced that number to four when working with severely brain-damaged patients. Interesting work can be accomplished working with two or three patients together, but this is not considered as group work *per se*, because with so few participants it is difficult to create the dynamics necessary for the members of the group to interact among themselves; the role of the facilitator becomes too central. On the other hand, if there are too many participants, the facilitator cannot observe the various interactions or correctly pace the group work.

Frequency and duration

Group work with traumatically brain-injured adults should be done on a regular basis, daily if possible. The length of the sessions may vary depending on the participants and the objectives, but we have found that 1-hour sessions seem to be a good length. Ideally, it should be the point of focus around which other therapy revolves but this, obviously, is linked to the constraints of the institutional setting.

At our rehabilitation centre it is logistically extremely difficult to set up daily group sessions over any sustained length of time. We face problems concerning the availability both of the therapists and of the room where group work is carried out. In addition, the average length of stay for our patients is 1–2 months. Our compromise, up to now, has been to have two or three 1-hour sessions per week over a 4-week period. That only gives us 8–12 hours per group, so our objectives have to be very specific. For severely brain-damaged patients, whose length of stay is longer, we can envisage groups over more extended periods of time. For example, our 'attention and concentration groups' can last for up to 6 months. Our 'stimulation group' met for over a year on a weekly basis. However, in these cases, we usually set up 1-month programmes, at the end of which we evaluate and adjust the programme contents, as well as including new members in a new month-long cycle.

Place

Where should group work be carried out? This is an important question, because, in order to do group work properly, there must be room for members to move around. Subgroups are often created and there must be enough space so that the various groups can work efficiently without distractions. On the other hand, the room must not be too large or participants will feel uncomfortable. The use of space is an extremely important variable, especially as it is very often an unconscious part of our cultural make-up [11].

The participants should feel comfortable in the room: lighting, texture, colours, movable tables and chairs are all points to consider. Ideally, it should not be the same room as the one where individual therapy is carried out. We have found that with groups of six to eight people in wheelchairs, it is best to have at least 50 square metres. If none of the patients needs a wheelchair, the size of the room need not be so large. Optimally, the space of the room should be modifiable, using large panels to delimit the space according to the needs of the group.

Programme contents and objectives

What can be done during group work? Objectives and subsequent programmes vary widely, but the basic questions to ask are the following.

- What can be done in a group session that cannot be done in individual therapy (be it physiotherapy, occupational therapy, speech therapy or neuropsychological rehabilitation)?
- How can the dynamics of the group be used to reach the programme objectives?
- How can each patient's experience be incorporated in group work?

We can only outline general programme objectives, as the actual contents are too varied to cover here. At our centre we usually have the following kinds of groups operating simultaneously.

'**Physical groups**'. We try to put patients together who have the same kind of physical impairment. In the past year we have organized the following types of group:

- 'upper limb groups' – patients in wheelchairs who have various problems using and coordinating upper limbs;
- 'preparation for walking groups' – patients who are beginning to stand up and walk but who have problems with their balance;
- 'wheelchair-use groups' – patients who need to know how to manoeuvre their wheelchairs in various situations;
- 'walking groups' – building up endurance and level of difficulty (different kinds of terrain, obstacles, pace) with patients who can walk.

'**Cognitive groups**'. This type of group can also be aimed at various levels, although it is obvious that cognitive variables cannot be isolated in real-life situations. Nevertheless, with these groups, we try to work more specifically on a particular cognitive strategy. In the past year we have organized:

- stimulation groups;
- attention and concentration groups;
- time–space orientation groups;
- current-issue groups (life within the centre as well as local, national and international events);

- memory groups;
- decision-making and planning groups;
- strategy and creativity groups;
- language and communication groups.

'**Social groups**'. These groups put the patients in situations where they must plan, organize and carry out a decision made by the group concerning some type of social activity. These have included:

- organizing an outing together – this can be culturally orientated, such as going to a museum, a theatre show or the cinema, or convivial, such as going out together for a meal at a nearby restaurant;
- planning a meal within the institution with the group members – this includes deciding on a theme and choosing a menu, going to the nearby market to do the shopping, preparing the meal, decorating the room and enjoying the meal together.

It is obvious that in real-life these three 'levels' (physical, cognitive and social) are inextricably intertwined. However, by setting up a certain type of group, it is easier to define primary objectives, even though we know we are working on several levels at the same time. A case in point to illustrate this is the 'social group' that organizes a meal within the institution. In order for this type of group to function smoothly, in addition to the necessary social strategies, it implies using all kinds of cognitive strategies (decision making, planning and organizing, remembering what needs to be or has already been done, etc.). It also calls for certain physical skills: going outside the institution to do the shopping, preparing the meal, setting the table, eating together and doing the washing up.

Currently at our centre, we are very interested in exploring this area: how to simulate real-life situations in a group task that requires various social, cognitive and physical strategies.

GENERAL GROUP ANIMATION TECHNIQUES: HOW TO CREATE A GROUP FEELING

After having outlined the preliminaries to consider in setting up group work, we can now turn to the subject of group animation techniques. Most of these techniques are inspired by, if not directly taken from, drama progression techniques [12–14], as well as communicative and pragmatic approaches used in teaching foreign languages to adults [15–17].

The first and most important thing to do, in order to have successful groups, is to 'create' your group. In order to want to participate in group work, each participant must feel comfortable, both as an individual in the group and as an integral part of the group. One way to create this comfortable atmosphere is to first 'eliminate the unknowns'. This can be done in the following way.

1. **Explain the 'logistics' of the group work**. Keep in mind the four general approaches to learning and be sure to answer the questions of who are the group leaders, why was this particular group set up and with what objectives, what are the programme contents and finally how will the work be done.

Make sure these four questions are answered clearly and simply at the beginning of group work. Explaining the logistics should only take a few minutes. This is not the time to go into lengthy discussions; the purpose is to give the participants a clear framework about the organizational aspects of the group work.

2. **Propose exercises that help participants become acquainted with each other**. Start to create 'links' among the various members. There are innumerable group forming exercises that can be done, but there are some basic rules to keep in mind.

- Do not put someone on the spot. It is usually a very uncomfortable situation when you have to talk about yourself in front of an entire group. Even just saying your name can sometimes be a stressful situation. Have them first exchange information in twos or threes.
- In order to avoid creating cliques, keep the participants moving, exchanging different bits of information with different people.
- Keep the information non-threatening. It can be personal but not intimate (e.g. something you love to eat, a sport you enjoy, a country you'd like to visit, etc.)
- Set up the exercises so that they are enjoyable but not childish.

3. **Get the participants to feel comfortable in the room where the group work is to take place**. Help them discover, and get a feeling for, the space in the room. This is essential, otherwise each person will stay stuck in 'his' chair and 'her' place. This will obviously limit the possibilities of interaction, as the same people will always be in the same groups and won't get a chance to work with others. It is usually possible to combine space exercises with acquaintance exercises, so that at the same time as the members are getting information about each other they are moving about the room. The group facilitator must constantly be aware of using the space of the room effectively depending on the proposed activities.

4. **Aim for complementary input by the participants rather than competition**. When working in subgroups, the context can usually be modified in some way so that each subgroup is doing something slightly different. For example, imagine a 'language and communication' group

where various subgroups are preparing a 'role-play' or simulation involving shopping. Rather than have each group prepare exactly the same sketch, which would result in direct comparison and competition:

- one could vary the tone (one subgroup is angry, another shy, another excited);
- one could vary the context (one group goes to the butcher's, another to the baker's);
- one could vary the roles within the same context (all must go to the butcher's, but one is snobbish, another a poor immigrant, another a hooligan).

Variety is unlimited, and these variations can enrich whatever point is being worked on as well as contributing to a relaxed atmosphere, because each performance is unique and therefore cannot be directly compared to another's.

5. **As a general rule, follow the progression from the individual to small subgroups to one large group and then back to the individual.** This gives each person time to first prepare his own ideas, then to compare and discuss his ideas with a few others, before discussing it as a group. If this progression is not followed, it is inevitable that in a group discussion the first person sets the tone and the other members usually follow the initial proposal. If there is a group discussion, it is important afterwards to return to the individual to give time for personal reflection or notes.

6. **The role of the group facilitator must be clear.** His/her role is to set the group up in such a way as to create maximum interaction among the participants and **not** between the facilitator and each individual person. Once the facilitator has given directions, he/she should generally not participate directly in the activities, otherwise valuable feedback information can be lost.

The role of the facilitator is to coordinate and observe, not to be the official judge who decides what is 'good' and what is 'bad'. Of course, a trained observer will note a wealth of information concerning the strengths and weaknesses of the various participants, but that information is to be used to organize the next part of the programme so that each participant can feel comfortable with his/her 'role' within the group. Each participant should come to terms with his/her weaknesses but also, and this is very important with brain-damaged patients, discover his/her strengths and remaining capacities and how to utilize them to a maximum.

The role of the facilitator is to help the participants discover that work and play need not be diametrically opposed. In order to create a pleasant, relaxed atmosphere the group facilitator is obviously a model: it is important to be enthusiastic and have positive intervention strategies.

During one feedback session, a patient said, 'In occupational therapy, when I draw, for me that's work. In group sessions, if the activity includes drawing, I have fun doing it.'

HOW TO ORGANIZE ACTIVITIES FOR GROUP WORK

The points considered under this heading are general pedagogical guidelines that can be applied to any learning situation. However, these points are all the more important to consider in group situations using an active communicative approach, because the variables are multiplied and must be carefully coordinated.

1. **Remember that it takes time to integrate information**. This is true for anyone, but all the more so for brain-injured patients. Learning is not a linear process, but rather a spiral one, done gradually and in successive stages. One can continually come back to an idea or exercise, but each time the context is slightly modified to introduce a new aspect, enriching previous knowledge (cf the previous example given concerning role play). This avoids boring repetition, but nevertheless gives brain-injured patients a point of reference, which they often need.

2. **Use a wide variety of tools and means**, but think about the logical progression and the dynamic linking of the various activities. Each activity should smoothly lead to the next, all part of a coherent, organized whole. Drama techniques and progression can be invaluable here. To continue with the role-play example mentioned previously: before doing the role-play, the drama progression would be (1) relaxation, (2) concentration, (3) imagination, (4) confidence, (5) creativity and (5) improvization. If this progression is respected and dynamically linked, the actual role-play itself is bound to succeed. If not, there is a good chance it will flop. In order for an activity to succeed, there must be sufficient breakdown and preparation.

3. **Inherent to dynamic linking is the use of preparatory exercises**, a kind of priming to prepare the participants for the activity which is to follow. Exercises can be done at the beginning of each session to get the participants in the mood for group work. Continuing with the role-play example cited previously, one could imagine starting the session by moving about the room in rhythm to some lively music and, when the music stops, greeting the closest person to you in a certain mood given by the facilitator (happy, bored, sad, tired, energetic, etc.). This exercise would prepare the participants for a later role play involving tone variation while shopping.

4. **Timing is important**. A competent facilitator must know when to change or modify activities, when to alternate rhythms, when to use music or silence. Correctly pacing group work is an essential parameter, but one that is difficult to master even after years of experience.

EVALUATION

What objective means can be used to measure the usefulness of group work? A quick perusal of the literature available concerning evaluation of group work makes one realize how difficult it is to decide on pertinent, objective criteria when attempting to assess the usefulness of group work [18]. One can use certain measures that are used in individual therapy: language tests (Chapter 15), memory tests, evaluating the degree of limb movement, autonomy scales, etc. depending on the objectives of the group. But are these measures the most pertinent ones when evaluating the effects of the group on each individual? How does one measure a smile or active participation? How can one objectively measure the building up of a pleasant, relaxed atmosphere with increasing confidence, toleration and trust among the various members? One can observe these changes within each individual, but we have not yet found a satisfactory means of evaluating these parameters.

Our solution up to now has been to propose both subjective and objective criteria, when attempting to evaluate the efficacy of group work. Participants complete self-rating scales before and after group work, as well as a questionnaire followed by an individual interview with someone other than the facilitator(s), i.e. one of the patient's daily therapists (physio, occupational, speech). We are not completely satisfied with this type of evaluation and are currently developing new evaluation tools (observation scales based on pertinent criteria to be evaluated).

TRAINING

Up to this point the focus of this paper has been on the group itself, suggesting how to set it up and some techniques on how to successfully coordinate the activities. A last important point to consider is the question of the qualifications necessary to be a competent group facilitator.

One need not be a trained psychologist in order to do successful group work. However, it is important to know how to observe, how to set limits, how to pace and calibrate, how to link activities, how to manipulate variables such as mime, body work, drawing, music, relaxation, imagination and creativity exercises, various role-playing or game-like activities, etc.

In order to feel at ease manipulating all of these variables, it is most beneficial if the future group facilitator has proper training. Being a competent facilitator implies knowing one's own strengths and weaknesses, before claiming to help others discover their potential. The opportunities for this type of training undoubtedly vary from country to country. If training in group facilitation techniques does not exist *per se*, another possibility is to look into workshops offered in drama–theatre departments. As mentioned previously, numerous group animation techniques are inspired from drama techniques. If it is not feasible to receive specific training, can you nevertheless attempt group work? If you take into account the guidelines set out in this paper and if you remember to propose exercises only in areas where you feel at ease, then you will undoubtedly have interesting and successful groups. Each new experience will give you increasing competence and confidence to propel you on to organizing your next group.

CONCLUSION

This chapter set out some practical guidelines in order to achieve successful group work. Difficulties in evaluating group work were discussed. Specific examples were given when possible from our experience, but many of the points raised have not one answer but many. Those interested in obtaining additional information are invited to contact the authors directly, but it is obvious that each reader must adapt these general practical guidelines to his specific setting.

REFERENCES

1. Schmieder de Munoz. *Rehabilitation Hirn Verletzter*. Stuttgart: Verlag W Kohhammer, 1974.
2. Fyon JP. Intèrêt d'un examen clinique télévisuel du traumatisé crânien grave. Réalités prospectives avenir. Unpublished Mémoire DES Rééducation, Marseille University, Gien, France, 1983.
3. Bérard E, Fyon JP, Delorme JL *et al*. A therapeutic approach of head injured patients through relationship: a test of psychodrama (playing a part), *Proceedings of the 9th International Congress of Physical Medicine and Rehabilitation, Jerusalem*. 1984: p231.
4. Bérard E, Fyon JP, Viale C *et al*. Approche pluridisciplinaire du traumatisé crânien grave en rééducation fonctionelle: la réadaptation par la relation. *Journée de Médecine Physique et de Rééducation*, Paris: L'Expansion Scientifique Française, 1984.
5. Bérard E, Emery JC. Suivi ultérieur des traumatisés crâniens au delà de la période de rééducation médicale. *Journal de Réadaptation Mèdicale* 1985; 5: 193–198.
6. Prichard D. Une approache communicative dans la rééducation de sujets aphasiques. In: *L'Orthophonie: approaches cognitivistes et pragmatiques. Congrès International d'Orthophonie, Isbergues, France*. Paris: Ortho Edition, 1988: pp206–215.
7. Plamondon J. A l'Hôpital Renée Sabran, Giens, France: Groupes de stratégie. In: *Propos de réadaptation – Canada* 1989; 8: 3.
8. Devin B, Prichard D. D'où la necessité de travailler en groupe. In: *Expérience en Ergothérapie: Rencontres en Rééducation IV, Montpellier 1990*. Paris: Masson, 1990: pp 23–32.
9. Thomsen IV. Late outcome of severe blunt head trauma: a 10–15 years follow-up. *Journal of Neurology, Neurosurgery, and Psychiatry* 1984; 47: 260–268.

10. Paillard J. Le Corps situé et le corps identifié. *Revue de Medicine de la Suisse Romande* 1980; **C no. 2**: 129–142.
11. Hall ET. *The Hidden Dimension*. Garden City, NY: Doubleday, 1966.
12. Stanislavsky C. *Building a Character*. New York: Theatre Arts Books, 1949.
13. Spolin V. *Improvisation for the Theatre*. Evanston, IL: Northwestern University Press, 1963.
14. Hamblin K. *Mime, a Playbook of Silent Fantasy*. New York: Doubleday, 1976.
15. Brandes D, Phillips H. *Gamesters' Handbook – 140 Games for Teachers and Group Leaders*. London: Hutchinson, 1977.
16. Way B. *Development through Drama*. Harlow: Longmans, 1977.
17. Polsky M. *Let's Improvise*. Lanham, MD: University Press of America, 1980.
18. Mager RF. *Comment définir des Objectifs Pédagogiques*. Paris: Bordas, 1977.

Developing communications skills: a group therapy approach

15

Janet Cockburn and Jacqueline Wood

INTRODUCTION

The ability to communicate our needs, emotions or thoughts to people around us and to reciprocate their communications is something that we take for granted. This ability is used as an indication of normality. Failure to smile in response to a familiar face or voice in the developing child, or to cry when hungry or wet, is an indication that all may not be well. Similarly, after traumatic brain damage (TBI), a verbal response is one of the indicators used to determine when a person emerges from coma. However, in the recovery process after severe head injury, there is often a long road from the first utterance to conversation that approaches that person's premorbid level. In some cases verbal communication may no longer be possible, and new communication skills may have to be learnt or little-used ones brought to the fore.

In daily life we rarely stop to think of the extent to which we rely on non-linguistic factors in communication and conversational interaction. Although conversation plays a central role in the life of most people, much everyday speech is essentially social interaction, in which the actual content is unimportant [1], and interchanges do not need to be spoken. The raised eyebrow or shrugged shoulders can be as eloquent as words. The intended meaning may also be different from the spoken words and conveyed by tone of voice, gesture or facial expression, such as a sharply expressed 'Thanks a lot!' to someone who has just hindered your progress. Argyle [2] noted that, although speech was the most characteristically human means of communication, much of human life was, nevertheless, carried out by means of non-verbal communication. He demonstrated that, where information from verbal and non-verbal channels was in conflict, the non-verbal was the more effective trans-mitter. Where information is not in conflict, understanding of spoken interchange in normal, everyday communication can be augmented by intonation, gesture, facial expression, repetition or recapitulation. These aspects of communication often violate rules of phonology and syntax, and yet enhance and enrich the intended meaning.

In most people, language comprehension and production is mediated by the left cerebral hemisphere. However, comprehension and production of the emotional qualities of communication may be mediated by the right hemisphere [3]. Even simple conversation also makes considerable demands on power of memory, inference and information processing. These cognitive skills are mediated by both cerebral hemispheres.

The neuroanatomical effects of TBI are rarely precisely located (Chapter 9). Thus aphasia, as seen after left hemisphere vascular lesions, is compar-atively rare [4]. Instead, severe TBI tends to be characterized by a general disruption of verbal and non-verbal communication as a consequence of cognitive impairment due to diffuse bilateral hemisphere damage. Parallels can be drawn between these dramatic changes and the more subtle changes in communication that occur in normal ageing [5,6].

In TBI, recovery of basic language skills often precedes recovery of the skills of analysis and synthesis that are necessary for successful communication and utilization of new information. Communication is thus characterized by poor understanding and responsiveness and may present as impaired ability to understand humour or ambiguity [7], difficulty keeping to one topic in conversation [8] or simply as inappropriate communication.

This altered ability to communicate can have far-reaching conse-quences. Relatives and friends may perceive it as a personality change, return to work may be jeopardized [9] and social adjustment may be affected for many years subsequently [10].

Traditionally, assessment of communication has tended to rely on formal measurement of impairments, using scales initially designed for use in aphasia following stroke. Typically, the patient is assessed in a quiet environment with only the therapist present. Treatment has also been traditionally carried out in this manner. There are several difficulties with this. Firstly, bearing in mind the very different pathologies in head injury and stroke described earlier, the tests may have limited relevance in head injury. Secondly, even where such tests identify impairments, these may only correlate weakly with ultimate handicap. For example, Penn [11] described a study in which two people were assessed at a test interval of 5 years, one of whom had a CVA and the other a subarachnoid haemorrhage following a fall. They were assessed on two scales – one measuring the structural aspects of language, the other the appropri-ateness of communication in everyday situations. Both subjects were 'chronic', being at least 2 years post-insult at the first assessment. Penn suggested that, by this stage, an aphasic person has learnt to make adaptations to the demands of their environment. Although structural aspects of language may remain unchanged, showing no improvement on formal testing, functional aspects become more suited to the communication context. This suggestion was supported by Penn's results with these two subjects. Neither showed improvement on standard aphasia tests but both showed some improvement in functional aspects, particularly in responsiveness to the interlocutor and in fluency. The younger subject had also returned to work during the 5 years between assessments. Both had received intermittent therapy during the 5 years, but their improvement was probably attributable to functional adaptation and use of compensatory strategies.

Finally, any improvement in communication within a one-to-one patient/therapist setting may fail to generalize to other environments. There are a number of possible explanations: other environments may be too noisy for a readily distractible patient and attention may wander during conversation (Chapter 11); the patient may fail to recognize the general rules of communication as such and may only apply any new communication skills in the therapeutic environment.

Acknowledgement of these problems has led to new approaches to both assessment and treatment.

A number of observer rating scales, which measure communication behaviour and the extent to which an individual has adapted to his/her behaviour have been developed [12–14]. Essentially, these rely on monitoring various aspects of communication during conversation. Videotape recordings of discourse were used by Erlich and Barry [14] to facilitate this.

Group therapy has been used in preference to individual therapy as it has several potential advantages. The main advantage is that it comes closer to a real-life situation than the artificial one-to-one interaction between patient and therapist, in which the patient is the recipient and the therapist the provider. Patients or clients at a similar stage in their recovery or with similar difficulties in social communication may derive considerable support from practising these skills together. They may accept feedback from one another more readily than from a therapist, who is seen to have no problems with the task in question. Role-playing can form a useful part of group activities, and real-life situations such as a discussion of a play or TV programme can be more appropriately presented. Additionally, opportunities can be provided for multidisciplinary input to the programme and evaluation of progress.

The published studies of group training for rehabilitation of communication skills after acquired brain injury have described programmes developed for out-patients or clients at a comparatively late stage of recovery [15]. This may be because it is not until this stage that failure to reintegrate into society or to return to work is recognized as being associated with poor social communication. However, there are arguments for commencing assessment and group training earlier, before the patient returns home and is exposed to the potentially distressing experience of a social situation with which he/she is ill-equipped to cope. It may be possible to identify such situations and practise them in the relatively safe setting of a small group in familiar surroundings. If there are only a few patients in a rehabilitation centre at any one time who are able to communicate sufficiently to benefit from such a programme, their opportunities for social interaction outside a structured group setting are likely to be limited. It may, therefore, be even more important to provide them with the opportunity to express themselves in an interactive environment and to play an active part in their own therapy.

Speech and language, memory and reasoning, awareness of rhythm and tone and the use of motor movements of gesture, are all involved in effective communication. These attributes cross traditional disciplinary boundaries of assessment, care and therapy and can best be developed by a combination of skills provided by members of a multidisciplinary team working closely together.

HOW TO USE A GROUP THERAPY APPROACH

Whatever the context in which group therapy is to be implemented, there are a number of common, basic conditions that have to be considered. The aims of the group in question need to be clearly defined. There will be considerable differences between a design appropriate for people needing to regain confidence in using higher-level skills of interaction prior to returning to work and one for people who are relearning that communication is a two-way process. Ideally, selection of participants needs to be planned with care and personal strengths and weaknesses matched so that meetings will not be a focus of conflict. Other factors that need to be taken into account are the size of the group and the frequency and duration of meetings. It may be possible to have short daily meetings with in-patients, whereas out-patient groups that have to consider distance and transport costs may only be able to meet once a week. Duration of meetings will be influenced by such factors as attention-span of participants, pressure from other rehabilitation demands, such as physiotherapy, and, again, time and distance involved in getting everyone together. A group may be convened for a short period of intensive practice of specific skills or may meet for several months with more general aims, where problems are extensive and progress is anticipated to be slow.

Levels of function should be assessed prior to the commencement of the group therapy and again at the end of the programme. As discussed earlier, assessments of functional communication rely heavily on observation of behaviours. This can raise questions of objectivity of appraisal, and the more structured the observational measure the greater the likelihood of good inter-rater and test–retest reliability. Although Hermann et al. [16] argued that the interactional nature of communication made it possible for the interviewer and evaluator to be the same person, it is nevertheless advisable to ask people who will not be involved in the day-to-day running of the group to rate progress. Objective evaluation, however, poses considerable difficulties. Measures of verbal fluency, or retention and recall of a prose passage in a formal test setting, may not show improvement but nor will they necessarily predict spontaneous performance in the outside world. Increased self-confidence resulting from practice and success is hard to measure on a standard test but may be the essential catalyst to improvement in functional communication. Observation of behaviour in a group setting, independent of the therapy group, may be possible but it is frequently difficult to set up apparently spontaneous situations in which the desired behaviours will be elicited.

Erlich and Sipes [13] evaluated the effectiveness of their group training programme by reassessing participants on the Communication Performance Scale at the end of the 12-week session. They reported significant improvement in several main areas, including topic maintenance, initiation of conversation and cohesiveness. However, variety of language use, which was one of the areas emphasized in the treatment programme, did not show any improvement. The topic showing least change was non-linguistic behaviour, such as facial expression, which was also the item producing the lowest scores at initial assessment. Erlich and Sipes, however, acknowledged that, as their scale was not designed as a standardized measurement tool, their data could only be considered as exploratory and more refined outcome measures were needed in order to provide a reliable demonstration of change. Sohlberg and Mateer [15], who described use of a similar programme with other subject groups, did not publish data evaluating the success of the programme, either for a group as a whole or for any individual subject. At present there remains a lack of reliability data for the measures available and a serious need for well-planned, well-run studies of group therapy to develop communication skills that are evaluated against the functional behaviours they are designed to improve.

DESCRIPTION OF GROUP STUDIES

In recent years, a number of exploratory studies have been carried out in the Brain Injury Unit, Royal Hospital and Home, Putney, London, with different group formats but the same underlying theme of using a group setting to develop communication skills of severely brain-injured people. These differ from other published studies, in that the participants are in-patients who have sustained severe brain injury and who can best be described as making 'slow-stream' recovery. We describe in detail two different approaches, discuss the advantages and disadvantages and suggest directions for future work.

GROUP 1

This group comprised four patients of widely differing backgrounds and aetiology. Their common link was that their level of social interaction was below the level of their basic comprehension and expressive skills. There were three men, aged 19, 20 and 45 years, and one woman of 55 years. All were resident in the Brain Injury Unit. Their premorbid intelligence level was assessed as average or above average. Two had suffered traumatic head injury, one a subarachnoid haemorrhage and one anoxic brain damage. All were at least 1 year post-onset. At the start of the study all were wheelchair-dependent, although one was beginning to walk with a stick by the end of the period of the study.

Functional deficits in communication noted in all four people by nursing and therapy staff included poor turn-taking, lack of initiation or maintenance of conversation, reduced sense of humour (excessive literality), reduced intonation and limited use of facial expression. Three of the subjects also showed inappropriate eye-contact. The fourth was blind as a result of his accident. Despite the difficulties presented by his condition for design and selection of material for group sessions, he was included because his basic verbal ability was well-preserved but he needed to learn and practise social, communication skills in order to make the most of his residual abilities. Group sessions also provided for him an important opportunity to feel himself still to be an integral part of society and less isolated by his condition.

This initial group was convened and coordinated by the senior speech therapist and the neuropsychologist attached to the Brain Injury Unit. Prior to the start of the experiment, the conveners each observed the four participants on two occasions, either in a therapy session or at a meal-time, and independently rated their communication behaviours on a 14-item scale, modified from that of Erlich and Sipes [13], scoring each item on a continuum from 1–5. The mean of the ratings was taken as the baseline with which scores at the end of the 3 months would be compared. Items with the lowest mean rating were: intelligibility, rate and rhythm of speech, syntax and repair.

The group met for 1 hour, once a week for 3 months. After this time the participants' progress was remeasured and the study was evaluated.

Themes covered in the group sessions were selected on the basis of the combined baseline profiles. Activities included discussion on what makes an effective communicator; verbal and memory games (e.g. 20 Questions, Kim's Game); other turn-taking activities, e.g. continuing themes; interpretation of intonation using audio tapes, videos of soap operas, etc.; topic discussions aimed at increasing functional vocabulary and improving syntactical and lexical selection. Feedback was provided mainly by peer comment, which had the advantage of being immediate, although occasionally insensitive! However, in general, criticism appeared to be received better from a fellow patient than from either of the staff members, and insensitive remarks themselves could form the focus of further discussion. Audio-taping was also used to provide additional feedback. This could be repeated as often as necessary and was useful for the conveners as a reminder of points to be developed in future sessions. Video-recording was not used to provide feedback for this group, because the one blind member would have been unable to benefit.

The final session was taped and subsequently used to determine post-treatment scores. Baseline and post-treatment scores were compared for each individual and for the group as a whole. Two participants improved significantly overall during the course of the group (Wilcoxon Matched Pairs, p, one-tailed, 0.01). The changes in level of rating were small, however and, although both people were over a year post-onset, the possibility of some continuing spontaneous recovery from initially very severe injury cannot be entirely discounted. There was an improvement in overall score for the group as a whole. When items were considered individually (Table 15.1), there was no significant percentage change for five items – variety of language use, topic, initiation of conversation, interruption and listening.

The items showing the greatest improvement in mean score were rate and rhythm of speech, syntax and repair. As these were among the lowest rated items at baseline, it could be argued that they provided the most scope for an increase in score. Also, as the assessors were also the group leaders, they were not assessing blind and were aware of the content of the intervening group sessions. Nevertheless, the changes suggest that the patients had learnt to some extent to pace their utterances, to use appropriate linguistic structures, to be aware that the initial message had not been understood and to make attempts to communicate it more effectively by some other means.

Some of the topics on which attention had been focused did not show overall improvement. Skills in turn-taking in role-playing situations, such as ordering meals or making conversational telephone calls, and proficiency in initiation or maintenance of a topic were no better, nor was there any indication that listening skills had improved. All the patients in this group had brain damage thought to include frontal lobe

Table 15.1 Percentage change between pre- and post-treatment total item score for pragmatic communication scale: Group 1

Scale item	Pretreatment	Post-treatment	% change
Intelligibility	11	15	36.4
Prosody/rate	10	15	50
Body posture	14	16	14.3
Facial expression	12	14	16.7
Lexical selection	12	15	25
Syntax	10	15	50
Cohesiveness	11	15	36.4
Variety of language use	14	14	0
Topic	12	12	0
Initiation	15	15	0
Repair	10	15	50
Interruption	12	12	0
Listening	13	13	0
Humour	15	18	20

lesions. Skills that involve responding to relatively subtle cues, such as changes in expression or intonation, are likely to be impaired following frontal lobe damage. Spontaneous speech production may be reduced or contaminated by perseveration and confabulation [17]. Frontal lobe damage may also lead to decreased flexibility, blunted feelings, lack of insight and egocentric behaviour [18], all of which may work against improvement in social communication.

Although the results from this study were limited, even the small improvements that were noted might be sufficient to make a substantial difference to the social acceptability of the speaker.

No formal assessment was made of generalization to social situations outside the group setting, although informal feedback suggested that initiation of any conversational activity by the participants remained low. In this situation, in which all the subjects were in-patients with limited independent mobility, they had few opportunities to practise social communication outside the setting of the group. However, they were not observed to seek one another out at other times, although patient A, who became independently mobile, would escort other patients, help push their wheelchairs or share his newspaper if asked. It is, however, an important part of evaluation that generalization should be measured, and one that should be incorporated into future studies.

GROUP 2

Whereas the participants described in Group 1 were all able to contribute to conversational interaction at the start of the study, there are a number of people whose spontaneous speech or motor output is very limited after severe brain injury, although they have some ability to make coherent and apposite utterances. They may benefit more from a group situation, in which the pressure to contribute is not solely on them, than from a one-to-one session with a therapist, in which they are required to concentrate all the time on input or output. However, progress may be very difficult to measure, because any changes are likely to be small, and the challenge to the therapist of designing and providing material for group interaction at this low level will be great.

The second group therapy experiment to be described was carried out with five very severely brain-injured people, aged between 23 and 64 years, all of whom were at least 1 year post-injury and had extremely limited ability to communicate verbally. Four had a traumatic brain injury, three as a result of a road traffic accident and one after an assault. The fifth had sustained generalized cerebral damage following hypotension. One used a Lightwriter as his main means of communication, although he could also use eye-contact and facial expression. This group was staffed by a speech therapist and an occupational therapist and it met for a half-hour session three times per week. The data given here refer to assessments at the beginning and end of the first 4 weeks. The communication scale used for this study differed from that used with Group 1. It contained six dimensions, each of which was rated on a six-point scale, with zero representing 'none observed' and one to five representing 'very poor' to 'very good'. The dimensions were: acknowledging–greeting; turn-taking; initiation; expressing emotion, by intonation or facial expression; clarity of communication (verbal or non-verbal); appropriateness. These were selected to provide measures of basic skills needed for awareness of self in relation to one's environment and for interpersonal communication.

Orientation in time, place and person was chosen to be the overall theme of the group. This was interpreted broadly to include awareness of own interests, experiences, likes and dislikes. Activities covered included introducing one another, complimenting one another, identifying characteristics they would like to change in themselves or others and characteristics they would like to keep. Strategies were also introduced to improve general orientation, such as identifying clues to determine the time of year. Simple musical activities were also used to reinforce initiation and turn-taking skills and allow for expression of emotion with minimal linguistic output.

Comparison between pre- and post-group therapy assessments indicated statistically significant improvement for four of the five participants (Wilcoxon Matched Pairs, p, one-tailed, 0.05, for all except patient G). Total scores over the group as a whole show an upward change for each item. It is encouraging that measured change should have taken place. However, in this group, as with Group 1, the assessors were also the therapists who ran the group and therefore could not be described as 'blind' to the proceedings of the group meetings. Within a busy clinical setting, where all members of staff have more to do than time in which to do it, it is difficult to provide a truly objective evaluation of ongoing activity by people who are not directly involved but nevertheless understand both the measures and the purpose of the study. It is, however, essential to a realistic appreciation of the effectiveness of group treatment of communication skills. It is also possible that much of the apparent change in patient behaviour could be due to increased familiarity with one another over the course of the group. Some functional carry-over to situations outside the group was noted, with participants spontaneously approaching and acknowledging one another, but incidents were few and no formal evaluation was made. As with the first group, these participants had little opportunity to practise the skills in an unfamiliar setting or with people who did not know them well.

CONCLUSIONS

The pointers from these two studies suggest that the potential exists for viable rehabilitation of communication deficits among severely brain-injured people by using group settings. Although repeated practice alone may not overcome the cognitive problems that underlie ineffective communication, the greater face validity and informality of a group situation may enable alternative strategies for surmounting a problem to be identified and reinforced to the extent that their use becomes habitual. Nevertheless, these studies represent a preliminary exploration of variables that need to be manipulated and controlled in order to measure the effectiveness of this form of therapy. A longer baseline would indicate the extent to which communication skills were stable. Evaluation of generalization into settings outside the group should be made. Follow-up studies of communication behaviour, weeks or months later, will indicate the extent to which skills were learnt and have been generalized into unfamiliar settings. The design adopted for both the studies described here is acceptable for exploring the viability of a change in therapeutic practices, but is inadequate for determining the extent of change in behaviour that can result from changing practices. It may be the only design possible in a busy clinical setting, but it will only provide partial answers. The need remains for well-designed and adequately staffed research, using objective baseline and post-treatment measures, to be undertaken in order that the preliminary indicators may be placed on a sound scientific footing.

ACKNOWLEDGEMENTS

This chapter was written while the first author was in receipt of a Research Fellowship in the McDonnell-Pew Centre for Cognitive Neuroscience at the University of Oxford.

We should like to thank Dr Keith Andrews, patients and staff of the Brain Injury Unit, Royal Hospital and Home, Putney, for their help and cooperation, and also C Wiseman, J Williams and C Pound for their advice.

REFERENCES

1. Cohen G. *Memory in the Real World*. Hove: Lawrence Erlbaum, 1989.
2. Argyle M. Verbal and non-verbal communications. In: Corner J, Hawthorn J, eds. *Communication Studies*. London: Edward Arnold, 1980: pp 50–61.
3. Heilman KM, Bowers D, Speedie L *et al*. Comprehension of affective and nonaffective prosody. *Neurology* 1984; **34**: 917–921.
4. Sbordone RJ. Assessment and treatment of cognitive-communicative impairments, in The closed-head-injury patient: A neurobehavioural systems approach. *Journal of Head Trauma Rehabilitation* 1988; **3**(2): 55–62.
5. Baddeley AD, Harris JE, Sunderland A *et al*. Closed head injury and memory. In: Levin H, Grafman J, Eisenberg HM, eds. *Neurobehavioural Recovery from Head Injury*. New York: Oxford University Press, 1987: pp 295–317.
6. Rabbitt PMA. Talking to the old. *New Society* 1981; **22 January**: 141–142.
7. Groher ME. Speech and language assessment. In: Rosenthal M, Griffith ER, Bond MR, Miller JD, eds. *Rehabilitation of the Adult and Child with Traumatic Brain Injury*. New York: F A Davis, 1990: pp 294–309.
8. Boake C. Social skills training following head injury. In: Kreutzer JS, Wehman PH, eds. *Cognitive Rehabilitation for Persons with Traumatic Brain Injury: A Functional Approach*. Baltimore, MD: Paul Brooks, 1991: pp 181–189.
9. Brooks DN, McKinlay W, Symington C *et al*. Return to work within the first seven years of severe head injury. *Brain Injury* 1987; **1**: 5–19.
10. Thomsen IV. Late outcome of very severe blunt head trauma: a 10–15 year second follow-up. *Journal of Neurology, Neurosurgery, and Psychiatry* 1984; **47**: 260–268.
11. Penn C. Compensation and language recovery in the chronic aphasic patient. *Aphasiology*, 1987; **1**: 463–474.
12. Prutting C, Kirchner D. Applied pragmatics. In: Gallagher T, Prutting C, eds. *Pragmatic Assessment and Intervention Issues in Language*. San Diego, CA: College Hill Press, 1983: pp 29–68.
13. Erlich JS, Sipes AL. Group treatment of communication skills for head trauma patients. *Cognitive Rehabilitation* 1985; **3**(1): 32–37.
14. Erlich J, Barry P. Rating communication behaviours in the head-injured adult. *Brain Injury* 1989; **3**: 193–198.
15. Sohlberg MM, Mateer CA. The remediation of language impairments associated with head trauma. In: Sohlberg MM, Mateer CA, eds. *Introduction to Cognitive Rehabilitation Theory and Practice*. New York: Guilford Press, 1989: pp 212–231.

16. Hermann M, Koch U, Johannsen-Horbach H *et al*. Communication skills in chronic and severe nonfluent aphasia. *Brain and Language* 1989; **37**: 339–352.

17. Levin HS, Goldstein FC, Williams DH *et al*. The contribution of frontal lobe lesions to the neurobehavioural outcome of closed head injury. In: Levin HS, Eisenberg HM, Benton AL, eds. *Frontal Lobe Function and Dysfunction*. New York: Oxford University Press, 1991: pp 318–338.

18. Stuss DT, Benson DF. Neuropsychological studies of the frontal lobes. *Psychological Bulletin*, 1984; **95**: 3–28.

PART THREE
Measurement

The principles and practice of measuring outcome 16

Alan Tennant and M. Anne Chamberlain

INTRODUCTION

Earlier chapters have described some of the challenges that have to be faced if the needs of those who have experienced traumatic brain injury (TBI) are to be met. Firstly, there are features associated with service delivery. The service has to be comprehensive and available to all who need it. Also, the appropriate service for a particular problem should be available in the right place at the right time. It has to be of good quality, accessible and, for those who need it, part of a comprehensive multi-disciplinary approach.

Within such a service individual techniques and therapies will be practised. Many of these have been inherited from previous practice or transferred from current practice in related spheres. Often there is little evidence of whether such methods are capable of producing the desired change. In many patients' cases we will not know how far change can be produced and will suspect that the benefit of therapy will be limited by permanent damage to the brain. Those practising in this area will be only too aware that, for some impairments such as visual agnosia, the apraxias and sensory neglect, there are few effective therapies currently available. One may turn with relief to a proposed new technique, but the practicalities of assessing its value (from funding onwards) are full of difficulties and may take several years. Yet, it is of the greatest importance that those responsible for providing care are in a position of knowing whether or not a treatment or a package of care is of proven benefit. We need to determine the outcome of treatment, and this means that we should have appropriate outcome measures. This is the focus of the remaining chapters in this book.

How do we select measures to quantify the impact of our treatment or the revised model of service delivery? Several recent books have summarized large numbers of available measures in general [1], in terms of quality of life [2], and for neuro-rehabilitation in particular [3], suggesting that often the problem is one of sorting through a bewildering number of alternatives. Richard Body and Maggie Campbell look at this in some detail in their chapter on choosing outcome measures (Chapter 20), but Shiel and colleagues also demonstrate (Chapter 19) that there are some occasions where existing measures fall short in their ability to measure changes we know to be taking place. However, before we address these issues there are some underlying principles of measurement, which we might usefully consider at this stage.

PRINCIPLES

CONCEPTUALIZATION OF MEASUREMENT

We have met the International Classification of Impairments, Disabilities and Handicaps [4] in earlier chapters, and it is described in more detail in subsequent chapters. Its value here is in helping us to think about what we are measuring, for the first principle is that we must be clear about the nature of the subject of measurement to understand the type of object we wish to measure. For example, pain (which is very difficult to measure) is an impairment effectively controlled by a whole series of discrete interventions such as drugs, acupuncture or transcutaneous nerve stimulation. Spasticity is another impairment that requires sophisticated measurement and technology, which will relate to the neurophysiological status producing the spasticity.

Disabilities exist on a different plane. A single impairment, such as 'mechanical impairment of the hand' involving, say, pinch grip or power grip, may lead to a whole range of disabilities, for example in writing or eating or dressing. The measurement of these disabilities is of a different order to impairment but nevertheless measurable in a standard way, and one example of this is given by Chantraine and Bérard in Chapter 17.

These impairments and disabilities, taken together, may then affect other dimensions of a person's life. For example, they may restrict the way in which a person can occupy their time or may lead to dependency upon others. These 'handicaps' are also affected by factors external to the impairment or disability, for example what support society gives to those who have disability, whether adequate provision is made for those with disability to engage in employment, and so on. It becomes clear from this that the measures required for impairment, disability and handicap are likely to be radically different and may well be addressed by different professions.

Identifying a conceptual framework helps us to clarify what it is we are trying to measure. We should make sure that we do not straddle the impairment–disability–handicap (IDH) boundaries in a single measure, and certainly not in a single subscale. Specifically, one should avoid 'scores' that result from adding together impairments, disabilities and handicaps.

VALIDITY

The second principle of measurement is that whatever we use must be valid. It must measure what it is supposed to measure; it must 'hit' the target – be that communication, mobility or quality of life. Ideally, one should use only those measures that have been shown to be valid, but there are many types of validity, and some of the processes have been described as 'part science, but to a large extent an art form'! [1]

Let us think of the way in which we would develop a new measure, for example a self-completed measure for one aspect of disability. Early in its development we might be concerned with **face validity** – whether the items that comprise the new measure are credible. This is one aspect of **content validity**, which seeks to make sure that the items selected cover the concept to be measured. We might enlist a panel of experts to help us with these matters or, as is more appropriate for self-completed instruments, go and talk with those who have the type of disability we are trying to measure, to find out what they consider to be the most important features.

We may well be then in a position to test the **criterion-related validity** of our new instrument. Generally this is done by comparing the results against some gold standard. Perhaps our new measure is shorter and easier to work with than another, which is nevertheless recognized to do the job well. Comparing the two (usually by correlation) would give us the **concurrent validity** of our new measure. Another way to provide criterion-related validity is to show that our new measure accurately predicts some future event; this would be **predictive validity**. As it requires monitoring for the future event, this is rarely done.

If no gold standard existed we would attempt a **construct validation** of our measure, which asks whether the measure makes, for example, clinical sense and produces the results we would expect. To confirm this we gather evidence using other types of validity such as **convergent** or **discriminant validity**. Here we might test our measure on two groups where we would expect the measure to show either a clear similarity (convergent) or a clear difference (discriminant). If our new instrument was designed to measure more than one dimension, we could also undertake **confirmatory factor analysis**. In other words, we would expect the items to group into the underlying subscales we were proposing.

In the end, we would try to provide the best validation of our new instrument that was possible; when choosing an existing measure we should look to see if that has been done. Outcome measures that do not provide adequate evidence of validity must be suspect.

RELIABILITY

The third principle of measurement is that whatever we use must be reliable. By this we mean that the measure can be used repeatably and, under the same circumstances, produce the same results. If we give a reference for a person saying he/she is reliable, we usually mean that he/she always does the job asked of him/her on time and in a satisfactory manner. Reliability in measurement is much like that and is normally measured by **test–retest reliability**. This is a form of correlation between the results taken at two time points on a 'stable' population. Finding the latter can be something of a problem. For example, in assessing the reliability of a questionnaire, one would not want to repeat the measure so soon that the respondents could remember their first set of answers.

Inter-rater reliability is also important; a measure should not vary depending on who applies it. If the variation between different assessors or interviewers is large, it may obscure true differences between patients. Beware of reports of inter-rater reliability that use simple correlation. For example, if one therapist consistently scored a measure 20 points above another, the correlation between the two would be 1 – perfect. Correlation is a measure of co-variation – how items vary together – but we are more concerned about the level of agreement, for example between raters. Look for, or apply, statistics such as Kappa or the 'Inter-Class Correlation Coefficient' as adequate measures of the level of agreement between raters.

Another aspect of reliability which is often widely quoted is **internal consistency**. This is based on the idea that underlying homogeneity of items (that is they are all trying to measure the same concept) is likely to give rise to a consistency in response. We often see Cronbach's Alpha as a measure of internal consistency, and a figure of 0.85 or above has become the accepted level of internal consistency. Sometimes **split-half reliability** is presented and is another way of looking at internal consistency. Usually the items are randomly allocated to two scales and we would expect, if they were measuring the same construct, to have a high correlation between the two halves.

SENSITIVITY

The fourth principle of measurement is that whatever we use must be sensitive to the change produced by the treatment. This may come to be seen as an essential part of validity (particularly discriminant validity), for it is saying that the instrument should be able to show a change in circumstances over time. Recently the 'effect size' [5] has been introduced to show how sensitive a measure is to change. Instead of looking at the crude difference between measures, as was often the case in the past, the mean score at time 2 is subtracted from the mean score at time 1 and the answer is divided by the standard deviation of the score at time 1. An effect size of 0.2 is considered small, 0.5 medium and 0.8 large, so the greater the effect size, the more sensitive the instrument is in picking up change. A positive or negative effect size simply reflects the direction of change and this will vary between measures. How much, one wonders, has the lack of proof for the effectiveness of much of rehabilitation in general arisen because the measures used had poor effect size?

EASE OF USE

The fifth principal of measurement, particularly when applied in a clinical situation, is that a measure must be simple and quick to use. A complex battery of questions taking 40 minutes to complete and requiring a particular type of professional is restricted to use:

- where 40 minutes is available, preferably without interruption;
- where the patient is able to cooperate for that length of time;
- where the professional is available.

Although such measures may have use for small groups of patients in a particular therapeutic setting, often the conditions for use cannot be met. If so, then the opportunity for comparison across patient groups, between professionals or between service providers will be limited.

Complex forms or scoring systems are less likely to be useful in busy clinical settings and run the risk of either not being used or being filled in badly. So, ideally the measure should have a simple scoring system and the logic behind it should be easy to appreciate. Relying on some 'magic number' appearing at the end of an opaque process makes it difficult for the practitioner to relate intervention to the resulting score in a meaningful way, and often this makes it difficult to generate any enthusiasm for measurement at all! This cannot be particularly helpful to the process of improving practice and, although such scores are often used to describe changes in groups, their use at the individual level is very limited.

CONCLUSION

In summary, it is important to demonstrate that the therapy on offer to patients with traumatic brain injury is effective, and that the measures used are valid, reliable and capable of showing change where we expect it to occur. Whenever measurement is done with clarity, economy and elegance, it will help to spread good practice, which our patients so greatly need.

REFERENCES

1. McDowell I, Newell C. *Measuring Health: A Guide to Rating Scales and Questionnaires*. New York: Oxford University Press, 1987.
2. Bowling A. *Measuring Health*. Buckingham: Open University Press, 1991.
3. Wade DT. *Measurement in Neurological Rehabilitation*. Oxford: Oxford University Press, 1992.
4. World Health Organization. *International Classification of Impairments, Disabilities, and Handicaps*. Geneva: World Health Organization, 1980.
5. Kazis LE, Anderson JJ, Meenham RF. Effect sizes for interpreting changes in health status. *Medical Care* 1989; **27**(Suppl): S178–S189.

Disability – the Functional Independence Measure

17

Alex Chantraine and Eric Bérard

INTRODUCTION

In rehabilitation medicine a valid and reproducible method of disability measurement is crucial. In previous chapters we were introduced to the International Classification of Impairments, Disabilities and Handicaps (ICIDH), produced by the World Health Organization (WHO) in 1980 [1]. After many approaches had been made to the measurement of the consequences of disease, the descriptors in the ICIDH provide a sequence underlying illness-related phenomena. They are presented as:
disease → impairment → disability → handicap
and are described as:

- **impairments**: concerned with abnormalities of body structure and appearance and with organ or system function, resulting from any cause; in principle, impairments represent disturbances at the organ level;
- **disabilities**: reflecting the consequences of impairment in terms of functional performance and activity by the individual; disabilities thus represent disturbances at the level of the person;
- **handicaps**: concerned with the disadvantages experienced by the individuals as a result of impairments and disabilities; handicaps thus reflect interaction with and adaptation to the individual's surroundings.

For a long time various scales have been available to measure the level of disability, and one of the first and probably the most widely used is the Barthel Index [2]. The Barthel Index was developed to identify the need for nursing care and as such is a weighted scale measuring performances in self-care (feeding, bathing, personal toilet, dressing, bowel and bladder care) and mobility (transfers, ambulation and stairs climbing).

In practice, no one method of measuring disability is obviously superior to others or necessarily appropriate for all purposes. For example, many assessment systems have been devised to describe the severity and extent of dysfunction resulting from different lesions of the central nervous system. As far as spinal cord injury (SCI) is concerned, they are all based on examination of segmental sensory and motor function. One of the most widely used systems to record severity of neurological dysfunction was described by Frankel [3]. More recently, detailed quantitative assessment systems for documenting motor and sensory function have been developed, including those by ASIA (American Spinal Injury Association) and by the National Acute SCI Study (NASCIS). These systems are too complex and costly for routine clinical use. For other neurological problems such as hemiplegia, the Barthel Index has been widely used. Other scales have been proposed, but none is entirely satisfactory for widespread use because some are too detailed, often subjective in their approach, measure social support rather than activity or take a long time to complete.

The importance of assessing patients at uniform times following injury or disease must also be emphasized when interpreting outcome studies with all assessment systems. Some systems are better than others for attaining repeated measures over the lengthy time of possible recovery from the disease or injury. Recovery is best assessed through repeated measures, using the same assessment system for neurological dysfunction.

Functional abilities can be assessed simply by recording the independence–dependence status of a patient's performance of important activities, such as walking, but reliable, quantitative systems for more detailed assessment of functional abilities have only recently been developed. The Functional Independence Measure (FIM) is such a tool and was developed by rehabilitation professionals in the United States. With its emphasis upon a mix of different motor functions, communication and social cognition, it is gaining wide acceptance. We will describe the principles of that new scale and report on an evaluation which has been performed by one of us (EB).

PRINCIPLES FOR USE OF THE FUNCTIONAL INDEPENDENCE MEASURE

A task force to develop a uniform data system for medical rehabilitation was established in the USA in 1983 to meet a long-standing need to document severity of patient disability and the outcomes of medical rehabilitation. The task force reviewed 36 published and unpublished functional assessment instruments, which were helpful in identifying items and rating scales that measure function. The challenge for the task force was to select the most common and useful functional assessment items and to decide on an appropriate rating scale which should permit most rehabilitation clinicians to assess severity of disability in a uniform and reliable manner.

The Functional Independence Measure was devised for this purpose. It assesses self care, sphincter management, mobility, locomotion, communication and social cognition. The data set includes, in addition, items that document patient demographic characteristics, diagnoses, impairment groups, length of hospital inpatient stay and hospital charges. Pilot, trial and implementation phase studies have been carried out since 1984 for the purpose of testing the FIM for validity and reliability in over 50 facilities in the United States. The FIM was found to have face validity and to be reliable.

The FIM is not intended to incorporate all the activities that would be possible to measure or that might need to be measured for clinical purposes. Rather, it is a basic indicator of severity of disability. Severity of disability changes during rehabilitation, and the change in FIM is an indicator of the benefit or outcome of care.

The FIM incorporates a seven-point scale for each item, which represents major gradations in independent–dependent behaviour and reflects the burden of care for disability. Burden of care can be thought of as substituted time–energy, which must be brought to serve the dependent needs of the disabled individual so that a certain quality of life may be achieved and maintained. The underlying rationale for classifying an activity as independent or dependent is whether another person, a helper, is required and, if help is required, how much.

The FIM is a measure of disability, not impairment. It measures what the subject actually does, whatever his or her diagnosis or impairment, not what he or she ought to be able to do, or might be able to do if certain circumstances were different. As an experienced professional, one may be well aware that a depressed person could do many things he or she is not doing, but nevertheless the person should be assessed on the basis of what he or she actually does.

The FIM was designed to be discipline-free – that is, a measure usable by any trained professional regardless of discipline. However, under some circumstances, some professionals may find it difficult to assess some activities. If that is the case, another more appropriate person can participate in the FIM assessment of a patient. If it is felt that only a speech therapist can assess the communication items, whereas a nurse is more knowledgeable with respect to bowel and bladder management and a physical therapist has the experience to evaluate mobility, the assessment can be divided among them. This is, for instance, what we do in Geneva in our ward meetings.

All items must be completed. To be categorized at any given level within each item, the subject must attempt either all of the tasks included in the definition or only one of several tasks. If all must be attempted, the series of tasks will be connected in the text of the definition by the word 'and', but if only one must be completed, the word 'or' will connect the series of tasks. For example, grooming includes oral care, hair grooming, washing hands and face, and comprehension of either auditory or visual communication.

Implicit in all of the definitions, and stated in many of them, is a concern that the individual performs these activities with reasonable safety. With respect to level 6 (see below), the question to be asked is whether the subject is at risk of injury when performing the task. A judgement has to be made and should take into account that there must be a balance between the risk of an individual participating in some activities and a corresponding, although different, risk if he/she does not.

PROCEDURES FOR SCORING THE FIM

Each of the 18 items comprising the FIM has a maximum score of 7, and the lowest score on each item is 1, giving a lowest total score of 18 and a highest score of 126. Those involved with the development of the instrument have been adamant in their conviction that a seven-level scale is necessary for showing patient function change with sufficient sensitivity. In the event, FIM scores are often rated higher during therapy than when the patient is observed on the ward or in his/her room. The usual reasons for this are the patient has not mastered the function, or is too tired or not motivated enough to transfer the behaviour out of the therapy setting. In this case the lower score is recorded, because this is what the patient usually does. There may be a need to resolve the question of what is 'usual' by discussion between therapist and nurse.

The social cognition items of social interaction, problem solving and memory are estimates of function in three important areas of a person's daily activity. It is worth mentioning at this point that, unlike the other areas of function assessed with the FIM, which have been in clinical use for years, there is as yet no consensus about the level of disability *vis-à-vis* social cognition. While the social cognition items have acceptable reliability, they have been refined as a result of comments made by users during the trial and implementation phases, and they will continue to be refined as more clinical and research experience is gained by the field.

DESCRIPTION OF THE LEVELS OF FUNCTION AND THEIR SCORES

- **INDEPENDENT** – another person is not required for the activity (**no helper**).

  7 **Complete independence**: all the tasks described as making up the activity are typically performed safely, without modification, assistive devices or aids, and within reasonable time.
  6 **Modified independence**: activity requires one or more of the following: an assistive device, more than reasonable time, or there are safety (risk) considerations.

- **DEPENDENT** – another person is required for either supervision or physical assistance in order for the activity to be performed, or it is not performed (**requires helper**).

Modified dependence: the subject expends half (50%) or more of the effort required to do the task. The levels of assistance required are:

  5 *Supervision or setup*: subject requires no more help than standby, cueing or coaxing, without physical contact. Or, helper sets up needed items or applies orthoses.
  4 *Minimal contact assistance*: with physical contact the subject requires no more help than touching, and the subject expends 75% or more of the effort.
  3 *Moderate assistance*: subject requires more help than touching, or expends half (50%) or more (up to 75%) of the effort.

Complete dependence: the subject expends less than half (less than 50%) of the effort. Maximal or total assistance is required, or the activity is not performed. The levels of assistance required are:

  2 *Maximal assistance*: subject expends less than 50% of the effort, but at least 25%.
  1 *Total assistance*: subject expends less than 25% of the effort.

EVALUATION OF THE METHOD

We would like to share our experiences in developing the FIM for use in a French language setting and, in particular, in a rehabilitation centre and in a brain-injury programme. Several events sparked off our interest. In 1989, Carl V. Granger presented at the international meeting in Montreal 'Functional Assessment and Program Evaluation in Medical Rehabilitation' [4]. This presentation introduced one of us (EB) to the FIM. At the time the instrument was being translated as 'MIF' (*Mesure d'Indépendance Fonctionnelle*) for French-speaking countries by Boulanger in Montreal, by Minaire in France and by Chantraine in Switzerland [5]. Also, in l'Argentière Medical Centre we had to reorganize a brain injury programme (BIP) and evaluate our patients. Previously, this rehabilitation centre used the Barthel Index. Several attempts to use the Barthel Index in the BIP failed, because it did not appear to accommodate the cognitive impairment produced by brain injury. Consequently, the difficulty of evaluating brain injury was highlighted.

The first goal was to become better acquainted with the FIM. The second one was to validate this new tool within a given rehabilitation team. Then we would have to use it in our BIP and assess its use in our rehabilitation programme to evaluate outcome independence. Several questions arose. How were we to become better acquainted with the MIF and to validate it within the team? Working with the booklet imported from the USA and translated into French proved to be laborious. Reading Granger's papers was interesting for those of us able to understand English, but even so, we did not find any accounts describing the application of the FIM in brain injury. The main difficulty we found was to have common and clear instructions to number every function as accurately as possible. However, neither reading Granger's papers nor working with the French written booklet gave us the details we needed. We therefore asked Granger's team for a video-tape of representative examples. The film was viewed by our team at l'Argentière Medical Centre, but neither the language nor the message were suitable to our French culture. Therefore, we decided to make our own film [6] and chose to use examples taken from daily life situation because we felt that these were the best guidelines for a functional evaluation.

The next question became: how do we produce a film representing practical situations in such a way for it to be a useful guideline for those evaluating independence in rehabilitation? It was clear that those having to evaluate must contribute to the scenario, for example physiatrists, nurses, occupational therapists, physiotherapists, speech therapists, as well as orderlies. Each brings his or her own feelings and experience to the situations, so that the scenes are representative of the whole team's experience. At the same time, creating the scenario must take into account the novice public, who must be able to recognize and assign a level of disability to their patients through viewing scenes from daily life associating genuine patients in their surroundings. It was also essential for the producer of the film to show the resulting disability rather than the impairment. It is more useful, for instance, to show a patient with a stroke illustrating speech disorders than to show a brain-injured patient whose aphasia does not necessarily lead to an overt disability. The requirement was for the producer to make a training video, i.e. a video in which each scene requires an answer in a form of an assignment. Each assignment would be corrected in the film, so that it provided feedback to the viewer.

Another question arose. Could the team reach competence with the FIM using the training video alone? The team had to go on evaluating patients in the field but at the same time to get feedback from the video-tape. The film had to validate the team's training for assignment. When should the team refer back to the video-tape? We opted to do so when a discrepancy appeared between the patient's behaviour and what would be expected according to the classification, and secondly, when a discrepancy appeared concerning a given situation within the team.

We set up FIM in our BIP in 1991. Patients with traumatic brain injury enter rehabilitation programmes at different stages, depending on local facilities. Patients can be admitted to some units early after their accidents and can be monitored in the same manner as they had been previously in the intensive care unit. Other rehabilitation programs start later on, when patients can participate in some activities of daily life. Before discharge, patients have to be evaluated concerning their real independence in daily life.

This gives rise to other related questions. At which stage is the FIM useful?

1. In acute care?

The answer depends on what one has to measure:

- to measure severity of the brain injury itself, other evaluation scales such as Glasgow Coma Scale [7] or the new classification based on computerized tomography of the brain are more appropriate [8].
- to measure disability resulting from brain injury, one can use FIM to divide patients into three groups:
  those having a score of 18, that is to say the lowest score, patients are then totally dependent and **cannot communicate**.
- those having a score between 19 and 25 are totally dependent, but **do communicate**.
- those having a score above 25 are **partially** or **fully independent**.

2. At a later stage of active rehabilitation?

FIM measures dependence in daily life activities (ADL):

- if the score is much lower than 80 (between 25 and 60), one can claim that the person needs continual care in the institution and is not able to get a weekend pass to go home.
- a score around 80 (60–100) means that the person only needs moderate help in daily life activities, even though there may be severe psychological impairment.

- a score between 100 and 126 (the maximum) means that the physical help is minimal or nil, but does not necessarily indicate social independence. To complement the FIM, it appears that one needs both a profile to appreciate the disability for social interactions and a scale to measure neuropsycho-rehabilitational consequences of the brain injury (such as the Rey-Osterreith Figure or the Neurobehavioural Rating Scale) [9,10].

3. To prepare and anticipate self-sufficiency when living at home?

- Scores lower than 80 are meaningful in this context as they are indicative of the need for help from an attendant to support ADL activities. Even with higher scores, some help from an attendant or carer may be necessary, because behaviour may present a danger.
- Between 80 and 100, in other conditions not involving the brain, the person should be presumed self-sufficient, with minimal help being required essentially for body care, 30–60 minutes, one to three times a day. For brain injury, such a score (between 80 and 100) is not predictive.
- Over a score of 100 a person is presumed self-sufficient. Again this assumption only holds true where there are no cognitive or behavioural disabilities.

Rather than using a global score, we prefer to use a profile for the FIM. These may reveal great differences between several categories, as illustrated in Figures 17.1 and 17.2, which show FIM in two brain injury programmes in Pierre Minaire's Rehabilitation Unit in St Etienne and in l'Argentière Medical Centre.

LIMITATIONS OF THE FUNCTIONAL INDEPENDENCE MEASURE

Can FIM measure the psychological burden for relatives? In our experience, it is only predictive if the categories 'social interaction', 'solving problems' and 'memory' show scores lower than 4. Such a score for social interactions indicates a heavy burden, but does not indicate how this burden will be tolerated by the relatives: FIM is not a quality of life scale.

Is FIM a handicap scale? Not directly, because FIM scores indicate independence or dependence in given situations, rather than overall. If technical aids can be provided, or if the particular situation becomes

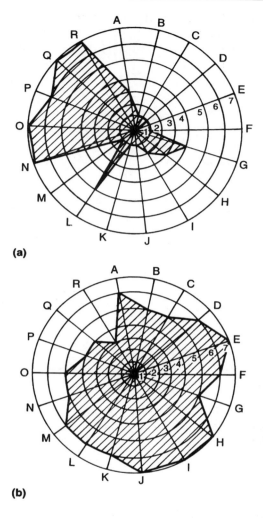

(a)

(b)

Figure 17.1 The same score may cover different realities. A functional profile is the logical component. **(a)** MIF/FIM score of a tetraplegic. **(b)** MIF/FIM score of a brain-injured patient.

more adapted, the disability may be alleviated but handicap may still be present because of other factors.

Is it reasonable to compare different populations of brain-injured people, using FIM scores? In our experience one can compare cases within functionally related groups, i.e. groups of patients having the same impairments.

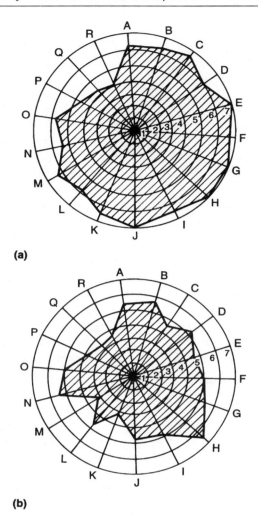

Figure 17.2 (a) Mean profile of seven head-injured patients (P. Minaire's unit). **(b)** Mean profile of 11 head-injured patients (l'Argentière Medical Centre). A = Feeding; B = Grooming; C = Bathing; D = Dressing upper body; E = Dressing lower body; F = Toileting; G = Bladder management; H = Bowel management; I = Transfer bed/chair; J = Transfer to toilet; K = Transfer to bath/shower; L = Walk–wheelchair; M = Stairs; N = Comprehension; O = Expression; P = Social interaction; Q = Problem solving; R = Memory.

CONCLUSION

In rehabilitation medicine, it has been emphasized that the desirable characteristics of any measure are that it should be valid, sensitive, reliable, simply communicable and relevant [11]. Among the numerous systems developed to measure disability, we believe the FIM provides the best information in many neurological diseases or injuries. Comparing similar global scores for subjects with completely different lesions or impairments has made it clear to us that the isolated global score without a detailed functional profile has little value. We must also emphasize that FIM is not a prognostic indicator and does not reflect the treatment required, but only dependence. Using the FIM in the BIP allowed us to identify threshold scores indicating that a score below 80 indicated continuing hospital care. However, profound disagreements emerged about thresholds above this level. One single social interaction dysfunction brings on dependence for all functions, and the resulting score of 90 signifies, for those in the BIP, the necessity of a person constantly present. A related criticism is that the FIM does not consider the psychological load which the patient represents for the treating team, although of course it was not created for this particular objective. Having said this, an important conclusion is that the FIM certainly constitutes a useful standardized international language tool, transcending cultural and linguistic differences, for use with those with brain injury.

REFERENCES

1. World Health Organization. *International Classification of Impairments, Disability and Handicaps*. Geneva: World Health Organization, 1980.
2. Mahoney FI, Barthel DW. Functional evaluation: Barthel Index. *Maryland State Medical Journal* 1965; **14**: 61–65.
3. Frankel HL, Hancock DO, Hyslop G *et al*. The value of postural reduction in the initial management of closed injuries of the spine with paraplegia and tetraplegia. *Paraplegia* 1969; **7**: 179–192.
4. Granger C. Functional assessment and program evaluation in Medical Rehabilitation. In: *Proceedings of Colloque International 'l'évaluation mesurable en Médecine de Rééducation'*. Montreal: Institute of Physical Medicine and Rehabilitation, 1989: p 23.
5. Boulanger Y, Minaire P, Chantraine A. *Mesure de l'Indépendance Fonctionnelle (MIF)*. Montreal: Sudmerr, Presse de la Faculté de Médecine, Université de Saint-Etienne, 1991.
6. Arnaud T. *Mesure d'Indépendance Fonctionnelle*. Vidéo film U Matic 26'. Sainte Foy l'Argentière: Centre Médical de l'Argentière Producers, 1990.
7. Teasdale G, Jennett B. Assessment of coma and impaired consciousness. A practical scale. *Lancet* 1974; **2**: 81–83.
8. Marshall LF, Marshall SB, Klauber MR *et al*. A new classification based on computerized tomography. *Journal of Neurosurgery* 1991; **75**: 14–20.

9. Stern B, Stern JM. The Rey–Osterreith Complex Figure as a diagnostic measure of neuropsychological outcome of brain injury. *Scandinavian Journal of Rehabilitation Medicine* 1985; **12**(suppl): 1–35.

10. Levin HS *et al.* The Neurobehavioral Rating Scale : assessment of the behaviourial sequence of head injury by the clinician. *Journal of Neurology, Neurosurgery, and Psychiatry* 1987; **50**: 183–193.

11. Sheikh K. Disability scales: assessment of reliability. *Archives of Physical Medicine and Rehabilitation* 1986; **67**: 245–249.

Handicap as a measure of outcome following head injury

18

Alan Tennant, David Hughes, Elizabeth Ward
Heather Warnock and M. Anne Chamberlain

INTRODUCTION

Recently in the UK considerable emphasis has been placed on audit – not financial audit, but the monitoring of clinical practice with the aim of improving that practice. A government publication called *Working For Patients* [1] placed emphasis on the development of a comprehensive system of such an audit covering local community and hospital-based services within our National Health Service – the NHS. Shortly afterwards an NHS Review Working Paper, entitled Medical Audit [2], defined audit as: 'the systematic, critical analysis of the quality of medical care, including the procedures used for diagnosis and treatment, the use of resources, and the resulting outcome and quality of life for the patient' (p 3).

The need to evaluate medical and health care procedures and to set priorities is vital to the allocation of resources from a limited health service budget, irrespective of whether this is a taxation- or insurance-based system. The use of expensive surgical procedures or rehabilitation programmes has to be justified in terms of short- and long-term benefits.

The advent of audit as an integral aspect of the measurement of UK health care services, particularly its emphasis on outcome and quality of life, has strengthened the need for adequate outcome measures. However, much of outcome associated with neuro-rehabilitation has a multidimensional nature [3,4]. Concepts such as 'quality of life' have yet to be both clearly defined [5] and seen to be relevant. The development of appropriate classifications and measures of these concepts is urgent.

Such measures should, preferably, be usable across disease boundaries and in a multidisciplinary setting.

In an earlier chapter, we described a project in which community occupational therapists (OTs) provided a community reintegration service for those discharged from a local neurosurgery department following traumatic brain injury. The community OTs used the handicap scales of the International Classification of Impairments, Disabilities, and Handicaps (ICIDH) [6] as a guideline to the domains that they should be investigating when undertaking a comprehensive assessment of need of patients recently discharged home. In this chapter we wish to describe how we used the handicap scales as a summary outcome measure, identifying the circumstances in which patients found themselves as a result of the interaction between their impairment and disability, and the physical and social environment within which they lived.

HANDICAP

The ICIDH is described as a manual of classification relating to the consequences of disease and concerns itself with loss or abnormality (impairment), restriction or lack of ability (disability) and the disadvantage (handicap) arising. In North America it is often referred to as the 'WHO' model or the 'Wood' model, after its author, Philip Wood. Its potential as a schema for measuring outcome is considerable, not least because of the multidimensional nature of its six handicap scales, shown below.

1. Orientation
2. Physical independence
3. Mobility
4. Occupation
5. Social integration
6. Economic self-sufficiency

Orientation is about an individual's ability to orientate to his/her surroundings, including seeing, listening, touching, speaking, and assimilation and interpretation of these functions. **Physical independence** reflects the level of dependency as measured by the frequency of help or supervision needed. **Mobility** concerns the ability to move around at increasing distances from the bed. **Occupation** concerns the purposeful use of time, including work, education and leisure. **Social integration** charts the individual's level of contact with a widening circle, from the reference point of self. Finally, **Economic self-sufficiency** is measured on a scale from zero economic resources to wealth.

These handicaps are all rated on a nine-point scale, with a tenth point for those who cannot be classified. The nine points form a clear hierarchical order. For example, as Table 18.1 shows, the mobility scale charts the degree of restriction that a person experiences, taking assistive devices and wheelchairs into account but excluding help from others. It ranges from being fully mobile through increasingly restricted mobility (for example confined to the dwelling) to being bedfast.

Table 18.1 The International Classification of Impairments Disabilities and Handicaps – mobility handicap

0	Fully mobile
1	Variable restriction
2	Impaired mobility
3	Reduced mobility
4	Neighbourhood restriction
5	Dwelling restriction
6	Room restriction
7	Chair restriction
8	Total restriction
9	Unspecified

The Physical Independence Handicap (Table 18.2) charts the frequency of help needed, ranging from those who are fully independent, through those who have 'long-interval' dependence (which is needing help on a regular basis up to and including once a day) to those with 'intensive care' dependence (i.e. the need for supervision or help continuously). So, for example, those with long-interval dependence may require only the provision of a daily main meal, whilst those with intensive care dependence may require nursing care throughout the day and night.

Recently it has become accepted that the interaction between resources, the physical environment and social attitudes on the one hand, and physical, psychological and intellectual aspects of functioning (impairment and disability) on the other, influences social outcomes or handicap.

Table 18.2 The International Classification of Impairments Disabilities and Handicaps – physical independence handicap

0	Fully independent
1	Aided independence
2	Adapted independence
3	Situational dependence
·4	Long-interval dependence
5	Short-interval dependence
6	Critical-interval dependence
7	Special-care dependence
8	Intensive-care dependence
9	Unspecified

Thus, although handicap was formally defined in terms of restriction of **roles**, experience with the use of these concepts has suggested that a more useful way of understanding handicap is to focus on the **circumstances** in which individuals find themselves. This way of looking at handicap highlights the need to give more attention to the role of the physical, social and psychological environment.

DEVELOPMENT

A prospective study, involving patients admitted to the Department of Neurosurgery at the General Infirmary in Leeds, UK from January 1990, has enabled us to examine short-term outcome following head injury. Survivors aged 16 years and over whose length of stay was greater than 24 hours and who resided within the city's administrative area were entered into the study. As well as relevant clinical data being recorded on a database in neurosurgery (a head-injury audit), patients were assessed as soon as possible after discharge by occupational therapists (OTs) working from a community base and the results were added to a therapy audit. The intention was to develop a fully functioning, coma-to-community electronic audit by utilizing the same software and to share data electronically between the different services. To date, this involves the Neurosurgery Department, the neuro-rehabilitation ward at another hospital and the community OTs.

During the first 21 months of the new service the median time to follow-up was 3 months. A comprehensive needs assessment was undertaken by the OT, using standardized measures like the Barthel Index [7,8] and the self-completed Nottingham Health Profile [9,10]. Outcome was summarized by the six ICIDH handicap scales. Occupational therapists assigned patients to the six handicap scales after an average 2-hour assessment. Assignment is undertaken in a manner similar to that utilized by the FIMS system [11], which was described in the previous chapter. This process includes functional assessment methods, typically used by community OTs in assessing physical independence and mobility needs, together with a range of standardized measures and checklists to help inform decision-making on the other dimensions. Thus, observation and extensive questioning allows the OT to decide on which point of each scale the client belongs. The ICIDH manual gives detailed instructions about assignment. For example, the scale point 4 of the Occupation Handicap is defined by the inclusion statement: 'limitations on the amount of time the individual is able to devote to his occupation, such as curtailment of recreation and other leisure activities . . . able to attend school only part-time. . . . able to sustain only part-time employment or occupation because of impairment and disability. . . .' (p 196). The wording of these scales is precise but not easily understood, so that the community OTs were introduced to the handicap scales in a series of meetings, and joint assessments were undertaken to establish interobserver reliability.

In our quest for making outcome accessible to managers and others (there are over a quarter of a million possible combinations of the six handicap scales) we developed a method of reporting the handicap scales by defining 'appreciable' handicap. This is scale point 4 or above on each of the six handicap scales. Table 18.3 shows what this means. Thus, for example, at the level of appreciable handicap a person needs assistance to orientate themselves to his/her surroundings or is restricted to the immediate environs of the home.

Table 18.3   The International Classification of Impairments Disabilities and Handicaps – appreciable handicap

Handicap	Appreciable level
1. Orientation	**Moderate impediment** (assistance required)
2. Physical independence	**Long-interval** (help once/24 h or less)
3. Mobility	**Neighbourhood restriction** (to neighbourhood of dwelling)
4. Occupation	**Reduced** (part-time only)
5. Social integration	**Impoverished relationships** (difficulty with friends, etc.)
6. Economic self-sufficiency	**Precariously self-sufficient** (benefits or other help needed)

RESULTS

We report here on the first 51 patients assessed in this way. With a mean age of 33 years (95% CI: 28.7–37.3), these patients stayed in hospital on average for 37.3 days (95% CI: 20.7–54.0). The mean Glasgow Coma Scale [12] on admission was 9.1 (95% CI: 7.6–10.6), reflecting the fact that those followed up are survivors of head injury discharged home. Over two-fifths (41.9%) were classified as having moderate or severe disability upon discharge, using the Glasgow Outcome Scale (GOS) [13]. Nearly a fifth (17.6%) had been discharged from the local neuro-rehabilitation facility.

Nearly two-fifths (37.3%) of those followed up were found to have appreciable handicap: 14% had one handicap, 12% two handicaps and 12% three or more handicaps. Table 18.4 shows the distribution of different appreciable handicaps.

Economic self-sufficiency and occupation handicap were the most common in the short term following head injury. Almost a third (31.4%) of patients were found to be dependent upon state benefits at the time

Table 18.4 Appreciable handicaps following traumatic brain injury

Type	%
Economic	31.4
Occupation	25.5
Social integration	13.7
Mobility	7.8
Orientation	5.9
Physical independence	5.9

of follow-up, and over a quarter (25.5%) of those followed up had appreciable occupation handicap – i.e. they were unable to return to their previous activity (work, school or homemaking) on a full-time basis. Other types of appreciable handicap were much rarer. Just over one in eight (13.7%) had appreciable handicap in social integration, i.e. they had problems relating to friends. Appreciable handicap in physical independence, mobility or orientation affected between one in 10 and one in 20 patients. The 10 combinations of handicaps that emerged are shown in Table 18.5.

Table 18.5 Combination of appreciable handicaps following traumatic brain injury

	Combination	%
1.	None	62.7
2.	Economic	7.8
3.	Occupation	5.9
4.	Economic and Occupation	7.8
5.	Social integration and Economic	3.9
6.	Social integration, Economic and Occupation	2.0
7.	Orientation, Social integration, Economic and Occupation	2.0
8.	Mobility, Orientation, Economic and Occupation	2.0
9.	Physical Independence, Mobility, Social integration, Occupation and Economic	3.9
10.	All six	2.0

The most common combinations are those associated with economic or occupation handicap which, either alone or as a pair, are found in 21.5% of patients. These two appreciable handicaps account for nearly six in 10 of all handicap combinations we observed in this set of patients.

Age ($t = 2.0$, $p = 0.052$), GCS on presentation ($t = 1.3$, $p = 0.203$) and length of stay in hospital ($t = 1.93$, $p = 0.066$) were unrelated to the extent of handicap as defined by the presence or absence of any appreciable handicap, although both age (older) and stay (longer) demonstrated clear trends. However, there was an association between (any) appreciable handicap and the Glasgow Outcome Scale on discharge, measured as good recovery or not (Chi-square 5.8, $p = 0.016$). As such, we found that the GOS was a crude but useful predictor of the time likely to be needed for assessment. The community OTs' comprehensive assessment took an average 82 minutes to assess those discharged with a 'good' recovery, whereas those discharged with moderate or severe disability took 156 minutes to assess ($t = 2.4$, $p = 0.026$)

The association between GOS and appreciable handicap is affected by the length of time to follow-up. When follow-up time is divided into two groups (those followed up at 2 months or less since discharge and those over 2 months), the significance of Fisher's Exact Test for association between appreciable handicap and GOS is 0.088 for the former and 0.383 for the latter. The trend is evident. The quicker the follow-up assessment, the more likely is an association to be found between GOS and appreciable handicap.

We also found a learning curve associated with the assessment, and thus the time it took to assign patients to the handicap scales. During the first 5 months of follow-up, when most of the effort was concerned with **how to carry out the assessment**, the average assessment time was 187 minutes. Despite there being no significant change in the proportion of patients discharged with moderate or severe disability (Chi-square 0.36, $p = 0.55$), assessment time fell to 98 minutes ($t = 2.23$, $p = 0.046$) for those followed up during the next 15 months, when emphasis was shifting towards **what to do following the assessment**. Membership of the community OT team was relatively stable across this first 20 months.

DISCUSSION

The need for useful measures of outcome has arisen largely out of the reforms to the National Health Service in the UK, with the need to cost and charge for each type of intervention. In addition, current UK reforms of community care services, with a switch in responsibility for those services to local authority (municipal) services [14,15] have led to a similar need for appropriate outcome measures. Thus outcome measures capable of being used by both health and social services will be particularly useful, especially where the two services need to work closely together, as in discharge following neuro-rehabilitation. Such measures should be capable of carrying clear messages to case (or care) managers about the likely requirements for care.

We believe that 'handicap' offers one such approach and that the notion of appreciable handicap offers a way of transmitting simple messages about the current state of the patient, and thus the needs arising. It is also ideally suited to a computerized database, which can convey a broad range of information about the client and their family based on a manageable amount of data.

Work is currently under way to identify the unit cost of patient care, both hospital- and community-based. This involves expanding the current database to include acute rehabilitation on the neurosurgical wards. We shall then be able to look at total costs in relation to patterns of appreciable handicap, shortly after discharge and again at 12 months. We will wish to examine how these patterns change as time passes and whether changes can be linked to different packages of care.

However, many questions remain to be answered about the use of ICIDH handicaps in this setting. Although we can see its potential as a summary of a patient's circumstances immediately prior to discharge, we are uncertain about its application in the hospital environment. How reliable will it be when many professions use it? Related to this, how extensive must be the associated training programme for using handicap scales in rehabilitation in general? Do we need to develop a training programme similar to that established for FIMS, with a training video similar to that reported in the previous chapter?

Certainly, from our experiences in the community we have identified the need to ensure reliability when new staff come to join the team. However, as long as a comprehensive assessment is undertaken (one which examines the issues related to each level of handicap), in practice assignment to scale categories becomes relatively straightforward.

Thus we feel that there is considerable potential in using handicap in this way but much still needs to be done. The fact that this approach is based on an international system of classification, which is widely used, is at least a good foundation.

REFERENCES

1. Secretary of State for Health. *Working for Patients* (Cmd 555). London: HMSO, 1988.
2. National Health Service Review. *Medical Audit*. Working Paper No 6. London: HMSO, 1989.
3. Kreutzer JS and Wehman P (eds). *Community integration Following Traumatic Brain Injury*. Sevenoaks: Edward Arnold, 1990.
4. Medical Disability Society. *The Management of Traumatic Brain Injury*. London: Development Trust for the Young Disabled, 1988.
5. Carr-Hill RA. Allocating resources to health care: is the QALY (Quality Adjusted Life Year) a technical solution to a political problem? *International Journal of Health Services* 1991; **21**: 351–363.
6. World Health Organization. *The International Classification of Impairments, Disabilities, and Handicaps*. Geneva: World Health Oraganization, 1980.
7. Mahoney FI, Barthel DW. Functional evaluation: the Barthel Index. *Maryland State Medical Journal* 1965; **14**: 61–65.

8. Cooper B, Shah S, Vanclay F. Improving the sensitivity of the BARTHEL Index for stroke rehabilitation. *Journal of Clinical Epidemiology* 1989; **42**: 703–709.

9. Hunt SM, McEwan J, McKenna SP. Measuring health status: a new tool for clinicians and epidemiologists. *Journal of the Royal College of General Practitioners* 1985; **35**: 185–188.

10. Hunt SM, McEwen J, McKenna SP. *Measuring Health Status*. London: Croom Helm, 1986.

11. Keith RA, Granger CV, Hamilton BB *et al*. The Functional Independence Measure: a new tool for rehabilitation. In: Eisenberg MG, Grzesiak RC, eds. *Advances in Clinical Rehabilitation 1*. New York: Springer-Verlag, 1987: pp 6–18.

12. Teasdale G, Jennett B. Assessment of coma and impaired consciousness. A practical scale. *Lancet* 1974 **2**: 81–83.

13. Jennett B, Bond M. Assessment of outcome after severe brain damage. A practical scale. *Lancet* 1975 **1**: 480–484.

14. *The Disabled Persons (Services, Consultation and Representation) Act*. London: HMSO, 1986.

15. Department of Health and Social Security. *Caring for People*. London: HMSO, 1989.

A score of zero?

Assessment of functional skills after severe head injury

19

Agnes Shiel, Sandra Horn, Martin Watson,
Lindsay McLellan and Barbara Wilson

INTRODUCTION

The patient with a head injury may have a variety of impairments which interact to cause functional limitation. There may be deficits in everyday skills, ranging from self-care tasks to those tasks which require differing degrees of alertness, information processing, planning and execution. Even when the patient is capable of using these skills independently of each other, e.g. of planning an activity without having to execute it, head-injured patients are frequently unable to integrate skills, that is to say to select and use the skills sequentially to solve real-life problems. The sequelae of head injury were described in Chapter 9.

Assessment of function is integral to planning and implementing rehabilitation programmes, but how useful are the well-known functional assessments for use with head-injured patients? Although it is necessary to use standard assessments in strict accordance with the administration criteria, nevertheless reliance on these alone means that some information vital to the rehabilitation effort is not collected at all. Levin, Benton and Grossman [1] have commented that 'data based largely on assessment of activities of daily living (ADL) lack sufficient detail to characterize residual social functioning, family relationships and recreational activities', which may be vital outcomes. ADL scales tend to share the common fault of neglecting the impact of cognitive deficits such as amnesia on daily life. It is possible for someone to attain a score within the range suggesting the capacity for independent living on the well-known and widely-used Barthel Index [2], for example, and at the same time have amnesia severe enough to preclude independence. Furthermore, it is not only important to know that the patient cannot carry out the task. It is also essential to know why he cannot carry out the task. Traditional ways of measuring functional status do not provide this kind of information.

When considering such terminology as functional impairment and functional assessment, it is useful to define what is meant by these terms.

There are numerous definitions in the literature, but the following two examples are representative.

- Functional **impairment** is defined as 'the inability of a person with an impairment to perform actions of a similar person without an impairment' [3].
- Functional **assessment** is defined as aiming 'to measure an individual's use of the variety of skills necessary to daily living, social interaction and other desired behaviour' [4].

These definitions have two major difficulties in the context of head injury which need to be addressed:

- they presuppose 'normal' or 'non-impaired' function, but give no indication of what this might be;
- functional assessments currently in use have a physical bias, which means that only one area of impairment caused by head injury is being assessed. 'Social interaction and other desired behaviour' is not measured at all, even though 'it is well recognized that for many patients the most persistent and disabling effects of severe head injury are affective, social, behavioural and cognitive rather than physical' [5].

In order to explain how functional assessment scales developed as they did, it is useful to look at their development.

Early assessments focused almost exclusively on measurement of the anatomical loss without cognisance of the effects of the loss. Hence, loss of a limb was compensated similarly for all employees, whether they were manual workers and unable to continue work or desk workers who could resume employment, and loss of two limbs was worth exactly double the compensation of loss of one limb, despite the fact that the functional limitation was likely to be more than double.

Following the second world war, a change in the method of functional assessment took place for several reasons.

- A large number of disabled veterans were returning from the war to seek employment and settlement in the community.
- The therapy professions were developing rapidly and beginning to produce their own assessments.

- Those involved in vocational assessment and retraining of these war veterans realized that the old anatomically based assessments did not answer questions regarding the person's suitability to live alone, to work in open employment, and so on.

Nowadays, there are a vast number of ADL scales available. Some focus narrowly on independence in self-care. Others are more comprehensive scales, including other skills and behaviours necessary for daily life. Some scales are better known and more widely used than others, and have gained reputations for being the most suitable tools for assessment.

One reason for the popularity of scales such as these is that they use numerical scores, which appear to be simple to interpret and to lend themselves to statistical manipulation. Most functional assessments use ordinal scaling, however, and this introduces a difficulty.

An ordinal scale is one where a progression of independence can be described but units of measurement cannot. These scales provide a rapid and useful method of characterizing a complex and multidimensional situation. An ordinal scale, however, is defined as such because the distance from one step to the next is not known, nor is it constant. Thus, adding values and then computing means, standard deviations or other statistics is meaningless. Consider the example of moving from the wheelchair to the bed in the Barthel Index:

Independent	15
Minimal help	10
Maximal help	5
Dependent	0

We do know that a change from 5 to 15 will represent progress, but these figures are arbitrary, and there is no reason to suppose that 15 represents three times the independence level of 5.

If summing within a set of items is problematic, summing across categories only compounds the error. If the score in this domain (which is mathematically meaningless) is then summed to the dressing score (which is equally meaningless), we arrive at a total which has no meaning in either ordinal or mathematical terms. If we progress to use this score as the level of independence and aim only to increase it as a total score, we may continue to fail to address the most critical problems of the patient. Furthermore, summing of ordinal scores may also mask improvement in one area and deterioration in another; thus a stable score may wrongly imply a static condition.

Some of the difficulties with using assessments already available with a head-injured population are as follows.

- Although they may indicate whether the patient can carry out a task independently or not, they do not indicate why the patient is not independent.

- These assessments have both floor and ceiling effects – if the assessment is used with a dependent patient who cannot carry out any of the elements involved, they are at the floor and therefore score zero, despite making some improvement. On the other hand, patients may score at the ceiling but still be very dependent, as with an amnesic patient who may get a maximum score on such an assessment but still require constant supervision [6].
- Such tests assess capacity (i.e. what the patient is capable of doing in a structured test situation) rather than assessing performance (i.e. what the patient will actually do when left alone with no prompting). Although structured prompts by a therapist may not be given, access to environmental prompts cannot be controlled. For example, if a patient in a six-bedded ward sees all the other patients getting up and dressing this will prompt the patient that it is time to get up. If the same patient was in a single room or at home alone his behaviour might be completely different.

In spite of these important problems with measurement scales, the scores continue to be used as if they have an objective meaning. Perhaps it is time to remind ourselves of the purposes of functional assessment – to see if these traditional measurement scales fulfil any of the purposes.

PURPOSES OF FUNCTIONAL ASSESSMENT

Why is it necessary to assess function? Roth et al. [7] have suggested the following reasons:

- to provide objective and quantitative measures of patient function;
- to describe and communicate levels of ability in self-care and mobility skills;
- to monitor changes in clinical status;
- to guide management decisions;
- to evaluate treatment efficacy;
- to prevent additional disability;
- to predict prognosis;
- to plan placement;
- to estimate care requirements;
- to determine compensation.

It can be argued that traditional scales fail on many of these criteria. They give a crude estimate of 'overall dependency' and are unable to provide sufficiently detailed information to monitor, guide or evaluate anything. Where is that information to come from? We would like to argue that it can, and often does, come from good clinical practice.

Leaving the last item on the above list aside, Roth *et al.* have given nine good reasons for carrying out systematic, objective assessments. All of them will be familiar to therapists, as will the notion that both the type and degree of functional disability must be specified in good rehabilitation practice. We set target goals and objectives, assess in order to identify problems, devise appropriate interventions and monitor progress. In good clinical practice, these are continuous processes and numbers do not come in to it. Therapists do not say 'Mr X scores 5 on dressing, and by next week we want him to score 10.' They might, however, say, 'Mr X has a problem with dressing caused by his weak left arm' or 'Mr X has a problem with dressing because he has difficulty in following a planned sequence' or 'Mr X has a problem with dressing because he does not recognize items of clothing.'

How have they determined the nature of Mr X's problem? By systematic observation, by putting Mr X in situations which sample real-life tasks, by setting up hypotheses to account for Mr X's disabilities, testing the hypotheses and using the outcome to specify the goals of treatment. We might measure grip-strength, degrees of flexion at the elbow or short-sightedness, and put numbers on these things to monitor progress and guide management and goal-setting, but we assess Mr X's skills, his behavioural repertoire, the things he can and cannot do, and the reasons for them by observation.

Observation is often regarded as subjective and therefore not as valid or reliable as a score on a formal test. However, there is little point in a formal test score that does not communicate the precise problem that will be the focus of the rehabilitation effort. Furthermore, observations need not be subjective and can be tested for reliability and validity. All that is needed is to carry out and record observations in a systematic, objective, consistent way. This systematic approach will include the operational definition of the activities under observation, and operational definitions of success, failure, degree of independence, need for help and so on.

An operational definition of a piece of behaviour is one which specifies the exact criteria by which the behaviour is judged to have occurred. For example, an operational definition of 'Drinks from cup independently' might be: 'Reaches out with either hand or both hands, picks up full cup, lifts cup to lips without spilling, drinks, replaces cup on table'. An operational definition of 'Drinks from cup with minimal help' might be: 'Independent as above, if cup is first placed in hand'. An operational definition of 'Drinks from cup with maximal help' might be: 'Drinks from cup if it is first placed in both hands and verbal instruction, "Pick up the cup and drink" is given, and helper steadies the cup as X lifts it'. Finally, 'Dependent in drinking from a cup' might be defined operationally as: 'Can drink from a cup when it is lifted to lips by helper and verbal instruction given to open mouth and drink'.

These definitions are clear and concrete. Any two people watching someone drinking from a cup would agree on the precise degree of dependence shown, and one person would be able to communicate it to a third person who had not witnessed it directly. The kind of help needed in order for the behaviour to take place would also be clear. Thus, the operational definition provides an objective and quantitative measure of function, describes and communicates levels of ability in self-care and provides a means of monitoring changes in patient status, evaluating treatment efficacy, planning placements and estimating care requirements. Because operational definitions can be precise and objective, they also allow inter- and intrarater reliability and both face and construct validity to be measured.

In the past few years we have been working with a group of severely head-injured individuals and attempting to develop a method of assessment which incorporates the principles of objectivity and relevance. In order to do this, we developed a set of criteria.

The assessment had to:

- **be concrete and behavioural**: i.e. a term such as 'dependent in transfers' would not be used; the alternative would be 'unable to get from bed to chair without assistance of one person to support left side, because of visuospatial impairment and left hemiparesis';
- **be operationally defined**: each element would have an operational definition, e.g. rather than 'dressing', 'can put on all items of clothing without any physical or verbal prompts';
- **focus on attainment**: i.e. we aimed at developing an assessment of functioning so that the aim was to identify what the patient **can** do rather than what he **cannot** do;
- **be timed**: we wanted to include some measure of the time taken to complete an activity; this is important because, if excessive time is spent carrying out an activity independently, the likelihood is that the patient will not do so at home;
- **take environment into account**: in some circumstances, patients are dependent in all activities because they are not given the opportunity to be independent – this is a different circumstance from the patient being unable or unwilling to carry out the activity, so we felt it was important to document which was the case;
- **be reliable**: this is self-explanatory – we wanted our assessment to have both inter- and intrarater reliability;
- **identify reasons for dependence**: this was the major focus of what we were trying to achieve; we wanted to be able to use the assessment to identify which impairments were proving a barrier to independence and where the actual breakdown occurred.

AN ALTERNATIVE APPROACH

We used a behavioural approach, which owes much to work carried out in the field of mental handicap. The precursor to this kind of assessment is Portage, designed for use with preschool mentally handicapped children. It is essentially a teaching technique, and the developmental assessment pinpoints gaps in functioning and thus identifies areas for treatment. It samples across a wide range of behaviours (motor, language, self-help, socialization and cognition). Items and goals are operationally defined, hierarchically organized and concerned with real-life skills. Most of the assessment can be completed by observation or interview with carers. Spurious numerical values are not used [8]. Portage has been used with neurologically impaired adults [9], but some of the items on the scale, which was designed for children, are unsuitable for adults.

The Hampshire Assessment for Living with Others [10] (HALO) and Bereweeke skill teaching system [11] use a similar approach, but with adults. They cover a wide range of skills required for everyday living. Bereweeke breaks down items into their component skills.

For example:

Component motor skills – drinking from a cup

1. reaching;
2. grasping;
3. lifting to mouth;
4. opening mouth on contact of cup and lips;
5. closing mouth to swallow;
6. setting cup down;
7. releasing cup.

A further example, taken from the goal-setting checklist for adults [11], can be seen in Table 19.1.

HALO also assesses how much help each person needs in order to perform the skills, as in the following example.

Feeding – Using a fork or spoon

Jack can grasp with a whole-hand grip with his left hand, but cannot use a pincer grip. He has some problems with coordination of his left hand and needs to be reminded to look at what he is doing. He has no functional use of his right hand and arm. He tends to neglect objects in his right visual field.

Jack's performance in the skill of using a fork or spoon has been described from direct observation. It is facilitated by the use of a fat-handled utensil.

Table 19.1 Item assessment and associated materials (from Felce *et al. Goal Setting Checklist for Adults.* 1986)

Item assessment	Materials	Performance
1. Grasps object	Apple. Place in palm	Grasps apple
2. Reaches and grasps object	Drinking glass. Place in front of client	Picks up glass (spilling allowed)
3. Takes object from person	Table fork. Hold fork out to client	Takes fork
4. Pincer grip	Toothbrush in holder or mug	Picks up toothbrush with thumb and fingertips
5. Gives object to person	Table fork. Give client fork, hold out hand and ask for the fork	Offers fork and lets go as fork is taken
6. Passes object a) 1 hand	Salt cellar. Place salt near client, point and ask him to pass it	Places salt near you or offers it to you
b) 2 hands	Serving dish. Place dish near client, point and ask him to pass it	Places dish near you or offers it to you

To be **fully independent** in this skill, Jack would have to be able to pick up the utensil, scoop, take the loaded utensil to his mouth, eat and set the utensil down with no assistance.

To be **fairly independent**, Jack would be able to pick up the utensil with a prompt about moving his head to locate it and a reminder to look at what he is doing.

To have **some independence**, Jack would be able to eat with someone to position the utensil and give verbal prompts.

To be regarded as having **very little or no independence** would mean that Jack could not or would not use the utensil. He would require complete physical supervision.

Jack would in fact be regarded as **fairly independent** because he can use the utensil but requires some prompting about its position and reminding about the need to look at what he is doing.

Note that environmental factors, such as the provision of an appropriate utensil, positioned so that Jack can see it, facilitate his independence to a large degree. These examples show the precise, objective, concrete nature of the descriptors. Anyone reading the account would understand the problem and the road to the solution. There is no ambiguity.

The value of systematic observation becomes apparent in the assessment of recovery after severe head injury, where patients may spend weeks or months in a state in which recovery is taking place but impairments are such as to preclude the use of many formal tests. In the early stages in particular, formal testing of the recovery of functions, such as some motor skills, cognitive abilities, social interaction and control of behaviour, cannot be undertaken because of the lack of appropriate instruments. Richardson [12] has commented on 'the paucity of objective measures of psychological function, which are sensitive indicators of mental processing and at the same time valid predictors of the ability to cope with the problems of daily life'. Wilson [13] has also drawn attention to the inadequacy of current methods of assessment, pointing out the poor relationship between performance on tests and performance in everyday life, the poor predictive power of formal tests regarding final outcome and the inadequacy of the information provided by formal testing for designing and guiding treatment programmes.

When required to use standard assessments of function, therapists are prone to qualify all 'scores' with further explanation to include the data that they consider essential. Assessment results frequently include such responses as 'needs help of one **but** . . .' or 'independent at this activity **when** . . .'. This method of assessment standardizes such observations. Assessing behaviour provides a system according to which where the factors affecting independence or dependence can be systematically checked, thus indicating where treatment efforts may be directed. It may also qualify results of assessments indicating the degree of support required by a patient. For example, a patient may be dependent because of severe physical disability but have few cognitive impairments. The help required by such a patient is very different from the help required by a patient who is severely cognitively impaired but physically unimpaired. A standard assessment of function would show the same level of dependency for both, but it is quite possible that the physically impaired patient could be left alone for some time, whereas it is unlikely that this would be the case with a person with severe cognitive impairment.

An advantage of this method of assessment is that, as the patient's behaviour is being assessed, it is virtually free of floor effects. This means that assessment may reveal change and can be used with benefit at an earlier stage than is possible with current standard assessments. If one can say that the patient can turn on and off taps, is aware of the danger of hot water and uses a facecloth appropriately, but cannot sequence these activities correctly in order to wash his face, such information would be understood by all, and it would demonstrate potential for improvement. Assessing behaviour may identify progress that is taking place but is not sufficient for the patient to change from one category to another on a less sensitive scale. The converse may also be true, i.e. assessment of behaviour may show that no improvement has taken place.

This approach provides a structured framework within which data documenting occurrences of functional behaviour, both productive and counterproductive, can be collected. Assessing behaviour can be undertaken simultaneously with assessment of disability – in fact, most therapists do this routinely, although not always systematically. In this way, the data generated by standardized assessments can be supplemented by such behavioural observations, which may answer the questions of why the patient is not independent and where therapy can be directed.

ACKNOWLEDGEMENT

This work was funded by grants from Remedi through the Wessex Medical School Trust (Grant No.309/22) and the Medical Research Council (Grant No. SPG8715555).

REFERENCES

1. Levin HS, Benton AL, Grossmann RG. *Neurobehavioural Consequences of Head Injury*. Oxford: Oxford University Press, 1982.
2. Mahoney FI, Barthel DW. Functional evaluation: Barthel Index. *Maryland State Medical Journal* 1965; **14**: 61–65.
3. Duckworth D. The measurement of disability by means of summed ADL indices. *International Rehabilitation Medicine* 1980; **2**: 194–198.
4. Granger CV. Health accounting – functional assessment of the long-term patient. In: *Krusens' Handbook of Physical Medicine and Rehabilitation*. 4th ed. Philadelphia, PA: WB Saunders, 1990, pp 270–284.
5. Brooks DN, Campsie LM, Symington C et al. The effects of severe head injury upon patients and relatives within seven years of injury. *Journal of Head Trauma Rehabilitation* 1987; **2**: 1–13.
6. Wilson BA, Shiel A, Watson M et al. Monitoring behaviour during coma and post traumatic amnesia. In: *Progress in the Rehabilitation of Brain Injured People*. Boston, MA: Kluver Academic Publishers, in press.
7. Roth E, Davidoff G, Haugton J et al. Functional assessment in spinal cord injury: a comparison of the modified Barthel Index and the 'adapted' Functional Independence Measure. *Clinical Rehabilitation* 1990; **4**: 277–285.
8. Bluma S, Shearer M, Frohman A et al. *Portage Guide to Early Education*. Wisconsin: Co-operative Educational Service Education, 1976.
9. Wilson BA. Adapting 'Portage' for Neurological Patients. *International Rehabilitation Medicine* 1985; **7**: 6–8.
10. Shackleton Bailey MJ, Pidock BE. *Hampshire Assessment for Living with Others*. Winchester: Hampshire Social Services, 1982.

11. Felce D, Jenkins J, Mansell J. *Bereweeke Skills Teaching System*. Winchester: Hampshire Social Services, 1983.
12. Richardson JTE. Outcome, recovery and rehabilitation. In: *Clinical and Neuropsychological Aspects of Closed Head Injury*. London: Taylor & Francis, 1990.
13. Wilson BA. Future directions in rehabilitation of brain injured people. In: Christensen AL, Uzell BP, eds. *Neuropsychological Rehabilitation*. Boston, MA: Kluwer Academic Publishers, 1988.

Choosing outcome measures

20

Richard Body and Maggie Campbell

INTRODUCTION

Clinicians and managers involved in head injury services now generally accept that the measurement of outcome constitutes an important part of the process that informs professionals and improves the service. What is less clear is how the desire to measure can be translated into practice. The purpose of this chapter is to consider the process by which appropriate measures are chosen to meet the particular needs of an individual professional, a rehabilitation team or a service planner, and to reflect adequately the change their treatment has brought about. We provide a practical framework, which guides the process of choosing measures but allows the reader to tailor that process to their particular circumstances and evolve solutions appropriate to them. It is hoped that description of the experiences (both positive and negative) of the team working at the Head Injury Rehabilitation Centre (HIRC) in Sheffield, UK will benefit other clinicians who are in the process of setting up outcome studies.

WHAT IS AN OUTCOME MEASURE?

It is clear from recent head injury literature that hundreds of measures have been used in studies that report outcome. These range from the broadest of global scales, e.g. Glasgow Outcome Scale [1] to highly specific tests of cognitive function, e.g. Trail Making Test [2]. Within published studies there are huge variations in time intervals, study samples, methodology, data collected and interpretation of results. As Brooks [3] points out, 'no one single definition (of outcome) is adequate for all purposes'. Therefore, when measurement of outcome is proposed it is essential to define what is actually meant by 'outcome', and a study of outcome should include a statement of the event(s) and/or process(es) the study is proposing to evaluate.

For the purposes of this chapter, the following broad definition of an outcome measure has been adopted: 'an outcome measure is an assessment or other recording that describes status after an event or at the end of a process'. This definition allows 'outcome' to be seen as a potentially fluid concept that is not necessarily limited to status at the end of a substantial programme or after a substantial period of time and can be directly translated into allowing the term to be used, for example, when evaluating a specific clinical intervention which may be time-limited. Within the definition there is room to consider such things as the outcome (or status) after 48 hours of a particular hospital regime, the outcome of a particular therapeutic intervention, the outcome at the end of hospital-based services, the outcome 5 years after hospital discharge and so on.

The breadth of the definition also allows the use to which an assessment or recording is put to determine whether or not it constitutes an outcome measure. For example, the Token Test [4], a measure of auditory comprehension, could be used simply to inform the planning of an intervention programme. However, the same measure, if interpreted in the light of either a particular intervention programme or the amount of time since injury, would constitute a measure of the outcome of the intervention or the status after time elapsed since injury. In the same way, the Glasgow Coma Scale [5], which is widely used to monitor the acute patient, can be considered a measure of immediate outcome of the head injury itself when used to assess status on hospital admission.

ISSUES IN CHOOSING OUTCOME MEASURES

If the end result of using an outcome measure is to be meaningful, then an appropriate choice of measure must be made. There is no substitute for careful consideration at this stage of the process. The desire to get on with the data collection in order to produce figures is usually strong, especially when there are external pressures (as when clinicians are required to produce data for management needs), but a lack of attention to the validity of the content of the measure or any other pertinent issues will lead to the ultimate failure of the project with all the associated dissatisfaction.

The project is more likely to be successful if thought is given to the following areas:

- project focus (or research question);
- choice of instrument (or measure);
- available resources (or feasibility).

PROJECT FOCUS

Why is the data being collected? What is it going to be used for? For example, is the data intended to assess the value of a specific clinical intervention or the global effect of a whole service? A gross measure of outcome may be adequate to document the overall effect of a service, but the same measure would not offer anything in terms of identifying which part of the service had induced any effect observed. There must, therefore, be a well-defined question that the data is intended to answer, and the measure that is chosen should provide data to answer that particular question.

Which group or subgroup of patients is to be the subject of the outcome measurement? The choice of appropriate measure is made much easier if the study sample has been defined in detail. For example, global scales and demographic data may be suitable for a study that involves consecutive admissions to a rehabilitation facility, in which the characteristics of individuals within the sample are likely to be extremely variable. On the other hand, a study sample that has a large number of features in common may prompt the use of highly sensitive cognitive assessments to measure the outcome of particular interventions. An in-depth single case study would present the researcher with a variety of other issues to consider, thus influencing the proposed data collection. Additionally, the period of time over which the study will run or the number of intended subjects should also be set, so that the study does not simply continue until everyone runs out of energy and enthusiasm.

Who will be using the data? Is it for the use of one individual discipline or is there value in collecting it in a form that can be understood by a variety of professionals? By considering this question before the choice of measure is made, one could avoid having to rewrite assessments and reports in order to communicate the findings to a wider group. The potential data may be of use only to those involved in direct care at the time of collection or there may be access to data that others involved in care at a later stage would find invaluable. This is an important issue in terms of continuity of care and integration of services throughout the lengthy process of rehabilitation and adjustment after head injury. For example, if all acute units were to routinely record the length and course of post-traumatic amnesia (PTA) using an instrument such as the Westmead PTA Scale [6], and the subsequent long-term outcome of the same individuals was documented, then the use of such a measure in predicting outcome could be assessed. In the absence of a baseline measure of acute status (such as PTA), any positive claims made in respect of the outcome of a rehabilitation programme may be left open to question. Likewise, an acute unit that does not have access to data in respect of the long-term outcome of those leaving their care cannot wholly evaluate that care or their choice of onward referral. It is entirely appropriate that individual clinicians, rehabilitation teams or managers of particular establishments should evaluate the effects of their own work, but it is also essential that they consider the value and potential influence of that work within the very much larger process of head injury rehabilitation in general.

When is the data likely to be used? If data collection is planned to continue over an extended period or if the data is likely to be of interest to someone making a retrospective audit, then the data should be recorded in a way that is not dependent on knowledge of current trends in terminology, etc. In summary, the focus of a project can be clearly defined by considering fully the use to which the data will be put, who exactly is to be studied, who will be using the data, when it will be used and under what circumstances. When the focus of the project has been identified, the specific aims within that focus should then be detailed.

CHOICE OF INSTRUMENT

The next step is to consider what data to record and in what form. An examination, at this stage, of existing literature and available instruments can help and may provide an ideal instrument for the purposes of the chosen study. It is important to note, however, that while there are many advantages in using validated instruments, such instruments do not exist for all the possible parameters of interest in the field of head injury. In addition, those that do exist have limited value in many areas of the service. It may be necessary, therefore, to search wider than the area of head injury, or indeed neurology, to find alternative measurement instruments that may be adapted to the particular question under investigation. Alternatively it may be necessary to design a new instrument.

What kind of data needs to be recorded?

There are a number of different ways of collecting data, each of which will have practical implications for the professionals contemplating their use and for the patients and their families. Objective measurements (e.g. range of joint movement as a measure of a specific intervention for the remediation of joint contractures) are likely to be relatively straight-forward to carry out and to have high reliability. They may, however, not be appropriate for measuring functional abilities. Many abilities are not realistically open to objective measurement and must therefore be assessed by means of rating scales, e.g. Functional Assessment Measure (FAM) [7], Glasgow Coma Scale. A number of practical issues arise from the use of rating scales, not least of which is the question of who should carry out the rating. Should it be carried out by one individual, by professionals from one discipline or by a multidisciplinary team? Rating by one individual may, in theory, be less time consuming but is vulnerable in terms of continuity, e.g. during periods of leave. Rating by multidisciplinary teams is often difficult to arrange, but may have useful side-effects in terms of team cohesion, development of knowledge etc.

The nearer any study gets to functional outcome, the stronger the argument is that ratings will need to be collected from the patient themselves and/or their carers. The well-documented problems of poor recall and lack of insight should inform the choice of rating to be used with head-injured people, and where possible the results should be corroborated. In addition, it is often difficult to get consistent access to the families and friends of people in rehabilitation, and their responses may need to be interpreted with considerable care.

Some ratings do not fit readily into well-defined clinical interactions, in which case a team may need to be inventive in its approach. For example, the FAM includes a seven-point rating of attention. A single score is required to represent a theoretically complex cognitive area, in which performance can vary considerably under different conditions. The HIRC approach to this problem is for clinicians of each discipline to use an attention checklist during their assessment, in order to inform the team rating of this item. The exact nature of the data to be recorded will obviously depend on the specific aims of the project. However, it is worth giving thought to the routine collection of a standard set of data, which can then serve as background material for a number of different studies. Indeed, some extremely useful studies of functional outcome are based almost entirely on this type of demographic data [8]. This would cover such things as data relating to pre-morbid circumstances and abilities, as well as information connected with the injury itself. Personal background data might cover age, sex, educational level, primary activity (e.g. employment, training, homecare, voluntary work), home circumstances (e.g. who the patient lives with) and socioeconomic status (though this is perhaps the most difficult to classify reliably).

The classification of even apparently simple items should be considered carefully. For example, it may be appropriate to record age at injury, at admission to particular facilities and at the time of administration of particular assessments or procedures, together with the time intervals between each of these. Many computer applications can calculate the intervals very simply from input of the dates themselves, thereby allowing routine access to informative data. One advantage of computerization is that the regular output and dissemination of data can stimulate consideration of whether that set of data meets the requirements of the study in progress. This is likely to be a lot more efficient than attempting to retrieve data retrospectively. A set of core information relating to the injury itself is more difficult to identify, as different establishments will require more or less detail depending on their place in the rehabilitation service. As an example, the data collected at the HIRC covers cause of injury, length of period of coma and ventilation, surgical procedures and drugs prescribed. While this data might not be sufficient for studies based round an acute neurosurgical unit, it seems appropriate for a community-based rehabilitation unit. It is relatively simple for this type of information to be passed from one unit to the next as it is factual in nature. One characteristic feature that makes demographic data easier to collect is that, once the original classification has been carried out, the data can often be collected by a wide range of people without too much danger of misclassification. For example, the HIRC classification of cause of injury covers the following:

- road traffic accident (RTA) driver;
- RTA passenger;
- RTA pedestrian;
- RTA bicycle;
- RTA motorcycle;
- fall;
- assault;
- work;
- sport;
- other.

Multiple entries are allowed (e.g. fall, sport would cover a horse-riding accident).

There are a large number of other possible systems of classification, e.g. the Uniform Data Set that accompanies the Functional Independence Measure [9], but this simple set meets the needs of the HIRC and, importantly, remains under the team's control should it need expanding.

It may be worth considering alternative methods of collecting the same data to allow as many options as possible. This would include telephone interviews (e.g. the Fone FIM) and postal administration of questionnaires, though Brooks [3] outlines some of the possible methodological problems that can arise. Obviously, all data collection will have to take account of unresponsive or linguistically impaired patients.

AVAILABLE RESOURCES

Having considered why outcome is to be measured and what information is required, it is important to recognize that the measurement of outcome is a potentially time-consuming and labour-intensive process. Before the final selection of measures is made, consideration should be given to the resources that are available for measurement to be carried out punctually, accurately and comprehensively. The number of staff available within any service will clearly have implications for the amount of data that can be collected, as will the time they can set aside for the tasks of data collection, monitoring and evaluation. Services that are under the time pressure of long waiting lists, for example, will need to set up structures that allow certain staff to carry out measurement, either as part of their routine clinical work or as a separate development. Failure to address this particular problem of time management could lead to such things as data not being collected at appropriate times, inaccuracies in recordings or staff stress (affecting service delivery or job satisfaction or both). Measurement of outcome also requires staff with appropriate experience, skills and qualifications. Clinicians who are suitably experienced would, for example, be able to make recommendations about the sensitivity, reliability, validity and clinical relevance of particular measures before they are put into use. They would also be able to monitor that they are being used correctly and evaluate results realistically.

Many skills (e.g. statistical analysis) may need to be brought in from other areas of the service (or indeed outside the service). Alternatively, training may need to be undertaken before the start of the outcome measurement process. Certain assessment procedures are accessible only to suitably qualified people (e.g. restricted psychological tests, neuroimaging techniques) and the availability of such individuals should be checked, as should their commitment to the project.

It is essential that the requisite experience, skills and qualifications are considered before any data is collected, so that services do not find themselves in possession of patchy data or data that they do not have the skills or time to interpret and put to use. It can be demoralizing for a team of people to put considerable effort into collecting data that then sits gathering dust. Where a team is thinking of collecting data over a period of months or perhaps years, procedures will need to be drawn up that cover issues like temporary staff absence (e.g. annual leave, vacancies), alterations to establishment (e.g. cost improvement programmes) and staff turnover. The service must be structured, so that it is possible for new staff to provide continuity of data collection sometimes within hours of coming into post.

OUTCOME MEASURES AT THE HIRC

Aspects of the process outlined in the first section of this chapter may be better illustrated by a description of the experience of the HIRC team in setting up the centre's first outcome study. This was not a problem-free process, but the experience gained may prove useful to other teams contemplating measuring the effects of their service.

The HIRC is a small purpose-built unit, geographically separate from the main hospitals in Sheffield, which provide community-based rehabilitation programmes for adults who have suffered traumatic head injury and who live within daily travelling distance. At the time when the process of selecting outcome measures began, it was staffed by a multidisciplinary team, including representatives from occupational therapy, physiotherapy and speech therapy, with occasional input from hospital-based social workers. When the question of measuring outcome was first discussed by the team, it was agreed that the major objective was to ascertain what, if any, changes occurred in the people who were admitted for a programme of rehabilitation.

ISSUES IN THE HIRC OUTCOME STUDY

The initiative to measure outcome came from within the team itself rather than being externally generated e.g. by health authority management. The project was, therefore, self-directed, allowing maximum freedom within the resources available. In considering how the potential data would be used, and taking clinical commitments into account, it was decided to collect a mixture of data that would guide, at least in part, the clinical intervention and include measures that could be readminis- tered to document any change. Thus, it was planned that the data would be clinically useful and also potentially suitable for publication.

Since the study was generated from within the HIRC team, this meant that data from other parts of the service could not be reliably obtained. Although there was, necessarily, a great deal of liaison concerning partic- ular patients transferred from one part of the service to another, the HIRC team had no control over any other part of the service, e.g. the acute neurosurgical unit, the subacute rehabilitation wards or the many surgical and orthopaedic wards to which head-injured patients were admitted, who in turn had their own (sometimes conflicting) clinical and service priorities. In addition, having a catchment area of six health districts, it would have been difficult to pinpoint, let alone negotiate with, those services that would be in a position to provide relevant data. The team therefore focused on aspects that were within its immediate control. Having what seemed to be one clear question, i.e. what is the outcome of attending the HIRC for a programme of rehabilitation?, it was decided to spread the responsibility for identifying suitable measures across the three main disciplines. The individual representing each of the professions assumed responsibility for those areas routinely covered by their professions in normal practice, i.e. assessment of physical function, communication skills and functional cognitive status. It was also decided to attempt to reflect the clinical approach of considering the whole person by including measures relating to as many aspects of functioning as possible.

An examination of the existing literature and available instruments met with mixed success. Standardized tests were identified for the measurement of cognitive function and for some aspects of communication. A number of scales attempting to measure global outcome were found, along with rating scales for behaviour and psychosocial adjustment. A previous search for appropriate assessments of physical status and performance in activities of daily living (ADL) had led to rejection of existing scales, on the grounds that they were questionable either in terms of reliability (e.g. grading levels of assistance), content validity or clinical significance, in that they did not assess why an activity could not be performed. An approach was adopted whereby the functional activities actually performed were recorded, either within a global rating scale or by means of an interview–questionnaire. The component skills and behaviours were commented on in other assessments, e.g. psychosocial functioning, physical ability. This necessitated the development of an assessment of the components of functional movement, which became known as Functional Milestones [10].

Although at the time there was no-one within the team who had computer skills, it was decided that the development of a database to record background data would both inform the study and be a sound development in clinical practice. As there was limited representation of professions, the choice of possible measures decreased (particularly in the areas of cognition and psychosocial functioning), and final selection of measures was influenced by the perceived feasibility of use. Another major limiting factor was the lack of published material relating to the out-patient head-injury population. The team (although small in number) had a reasonable level of experience in the area of head-injury rehabilitation, but still found it necessary in the end to make some choices on the basis of 'an educated guess' and others for a 'trial' period in the first instance.

The original study ran from November 1988 until early 1990 (and a revamped version until late 1990) and included all the individuals admitted to the centre during that period. Measures included two global outcome scales, recording of demographic data, a battery of cognitive tests, an assessment of physical function, a test of psychosocial adjustment and a behavioural rating scale. By the time the amended version was under way the demographic data recording had expanded, the functional physical assessment had developed and some of the cognitive tests were still being used. The global outcome measures had been replaced by semi-structured questionnaires involving the patient and carer. What follows is an overview of the positive and negative aspects of the original approach.

REVIEW OF HIRC OUTCOME STUDY

The basic idea of combining clinical and research needs had a positive effect on clinical practice, in terms of evaluation and development of clinical intervention and, in particular, in forging the development of real integrated team working. It also, as a byproduct, defined minimum standards of assessment. The negative aspects of combining clinical and research needs tended to be to the detriment of the formal research process, but this was related more to the issue of resources rather than to the approach.

In deciding to concentrate on aspects that were within the team's immediate control, it was possible to make adaptations quickly, and the data collected was, in the main, immediately relevant to the collectors. A negative result of this decision was the lack of hard data referring to the acute stage and, in particular, information that would inform the question of severity of injury. Also, because the project was happening in isolation from other parts of the service, the potential for a wider group to adapt their practice in the light of the findings was lost. It became clear early on in the process that what had been assumed to be one relatively simple question was, in fact, a complex composite question. In addition, as each individual discipline had taken responsibility for identifying suitable instruments to measure their particular 'speciality', the question had been interpreted differently and to different degrees. A vital part of the process, i.e. defining specific aims following the identification of a more general focus, had been missed because workers in each discipline assumed that they were of one mind with the others and, perhaps more importantly, were too polite to question each other about what exactly they were proposing to do.

Although the 'discipline-specific' assessments were generally completed at the appropriate times, it was more difficult to achieve continuity in the completion of those assessments, reflecting areas that the disciplines did not traditionally have responsibility for. This, again, related to a problem of resources, in that as demand for the service increased, the research aspect was less easy to preserve. The process of extra clinical workload, impinging on time mentally allocated to research, was an insidious one and was difficult to halt, given that the research initiative had come from the clinicians. Although managers were supportive in spirit, they could not provide the increase in staff that would have allowed successful continuation of the project.

At the planning stage there had been discussion regarding the timing of measurements, and it was decided to target admission and discharge rather than specific periods post-injury, since this would theoretically coincide with the team's own need to plan clinical input. Since there was no coordinated service for patients to be referred on to after discharge from the unit, it was also felt that the team had a responsibility to assess status at some point after discharge, and an initial target of 6- and 12-month follow-up was set. It was felt that this would contribute to a more complete picture of patients' progress over a realistic period of time. Although this was theoretically sound, it was found that in addition to increasing the overall workload, it had the effect of raising some patients' expectations of either a resumption of input or referral to a suitable agency for any new problem which might have arisen since discharge.

One major planning error in the area of resources was not considering the additional time required to properly collate the data and prepare it in a form suitable for publication. Continuation of the study became increasingly difficult during a period of rapidly increasing demand for the clinical service and ground to a complete halt when the occupational therapy member of the team left and the vacancy was frozen for a time.

Review of assessments

A very positive aspect of the whole process was the identification of those instruments that were and were not useful for the population in question. From that process the team was able to develop a critical perspective on the wider subject of measurement of outcome. Some of the issues that arose from the use of specific measures are detailed below.

It should be borne in mind that these issues arose in relation to a client group that was undergoing community rehabilitation. Inherent in global assessments is a specific set of problems that centres on attempting to achieve a balance between the comprehensive measurement of all relevant areas, sensitivity to change, ease of administration and reliability. For this reason, the team experimented with several measures to allow comparison of their strengths and weaknesses.

The Disability Rating Scale [11] was found to be easy to complete and to have high reliability, but did not provide sensitive enough information at the higher-functioning end of the scale.

The Glasgow Assessment Schedule (GAS) [12] documented a wider range of problems, but was felt to place too much reliance on self-report, the accuracy of which can be confounded by lack of insight or denial. Corroborative evidence from relatives often proved difficult to obtain, and discrepancies in reporting difficult to reconcile. Recent experimentation with the FAM has revealed certain limitations that seem to affect many scales (e.g. too low a ceiling on certain items to represent freedom from functional problems), but there are enough positive features to warrant further investigation. These include the detailed scoring definitions that accompany each point of each subscale and the expansion from the original FIM to include aspects of functioning relevant to brain injury (i.e. cognitive and psychosocial functioning).

Lack of sensitivity to either high-level abilities or the functional application of those abilities is not limited to global assessments. Some tests of cognition are specifically aimed at functional skills, e.g. Rivermead Behavioural Memory Test (RBMT) [13] and Chessington Occupational Therapy Neurological Assessment Battery (COTNAB) [14], but still do not provide a picture of how those skills are applied in the community. This is not necessarily a limitation of the tests themselves but may be an argument for combining them with questionnaires, checklists etc. to provide an overall picture.

Because of the fact that they purposely attempt to isolate particular cognitive skills, the 'pure' cognitive tests were found to document change in only a small percentage of the group being studied. Many tests of communication, for example, were originally designed for use with the stroke population and were found to be of limited applicability in head-injury (Chapter 15). The need for them to be administered under controlled conditions limited their flexibility, as did the fact that most are subject to well-defined test–retest intervals, which made them difficult to coordinate with preset outcome assessment intervals (i.e. admission and discharge).

One further unpredicted complication of cognitive tests was that it proved impossible to monitor, let alone control, the use of the same tests by professionals in other parts of the service or other districts (and/or their students). This meant that interpretation of any data was obscured by possible learning effects. As a result of these restrictions, it may be that 'pure' cognitive assessments are best suited to measurement of outcome of specific interventions with carefully selected study samples rather than as routine outcome measures on broad groups.

The approach of assessing components of functional movement seemed clinically relevant and functionally useful, and the assessment developed at the centre did not experience the same problems of high level ceiling or feasibility of use, since its original development criteria covered both of these areas. The use of what had been loosely termed 'background data' at the beginning of the study took on increasing importance. It became apparent, for example, that the category relating to the patient's home circumstances (i.e. who shared their living accommodation) was a sensitive indicator of many other factors, such as behaviour and independence, notwithstanding the need to keep external factors (e.g. natural chronological progression within families) in mind when interpreting the data.

The experiences of the first study and the addition of extra staff (including permanent clinical psychology and social work input) have helped the team to outline specific questions about outcome on which to base data collection. Currently the measurement of outcome of the broad group attending for rehabilitation includes a wide range of personal and injury-related data, together with rating on the FAM at admission and discharge. Assessments of specific skills are used to evaluate and plan intervention and to evaluate individual outcomes.

A separate study involves the use of assessments of family interaction, the focus for this having been set by a recent grant to improve the services to relatives.

SUMMARY

As well as supplying information about the effectiveness of head injury care, the measurement of outcome can serve to facilitate cohesion across disparate services and increase understanding of the exact nature of particular assessments. The process of setting up and attempting to carry out a broad outcome study at the HIRC has highlighted a number of issues that apply to the measurement of outcome in general. These relate, specifically, to the need to define in detail the aims of any outcome study, to select measures carefully that will meet the aims and to consider all the resource implications before any data is collected.

REFERENCES

1. Jennett B, Bond M. Assessment of outcome after severe brain damage. *Lancet* 1982; **1**: 480–487.
2. Reitan RM, Davison LA. *Clinical Neuro-Psychology: Current Status and Applications*. New York: Hemisphere, 1974.
3. Brooks N. Defining outcome. *Brain Injury* 1989; **3**: 325–329.
4. DeRenzi E, Faglioni P. Normative data and screening power of a shortened version of the Token Test. *Cortex* 1978; **14**: 41–49.
5. Teasdale G, Jennett B. Assessment of coma and impaired consciousness: a practical scale. *Lancet* 1974; **ii**: 81–84.
6. Shores RS, Marosszeky JE, Sandanam J et al. Preliminary validation of a clinical scale for measuring the duration of post-traumatic amnesia. *Medical Journal of Australia* 1986; **144**: 569–572.
7. Santa Clara Valley Medical Center. Functional Assessment Measure (unpublished). 751 South Bascom Avenue, San José, CA 95128.
8. Cope DN, Cole JR, Hall KM et al. Brain injury: analysis of outcome in a post-acute rehabilitation system. *Brain Injury* 1991; **5**: 111–125.
9. State University of New York. *Uniform Data Set for Medical Rehabilitation and Functional Independence Measure*. Version 3.0. Buffalo, NY: SUNY, 1990.
10. Campbell M. Functional milestones; assessment of physical function in the adult post head-injury (unpublished). Head Injury Rehabilitation Centre, Albert Terrace Road, Sheffield.
11. Rappaport M, Hall KM, Hopkins HK. Disability Rating Scale for severe head trauma: coma to community. *Archives of Physical Medicine and Rehabilitation* 1982; **63**: 118–123.

12. Livingston MG, Livingston HM. The Glasgow Assessment Schedule: clinical and research assessment of head injury outcome. *International Rehabilitation Medicine* 1985; **7**: 145–149.
13. Wilson B, Cockburn J, Baddeley ADB. *The Rivermead Behavioural Memory Test Manual*. Titchfield: Thames Valley Test Company, PO14 4AF, 1985.
14. Tyerman R, Tyerman A, Howard P *et al. The Chessington Occupational Therapy Neurological Assessment Battery*. Nottingham: Nottingham Rehabilitation Limited, 1986.

PART FOUR
Reflections

M.Anne Chamberlain, Vera C. Neumann
and Alan Tennant

In this book we have aimed to present the reader with some of the more important, newer ideas about the treatment, service structure and measurement of outcome following traumatic brain injury. We are all aware of the wide variation in provision and practice across Europe, but believe that, although treatment innovations in well-resourced countries may seem inappropriate, at least in the short term, for less well-resourced countries they may yet offer a basis for development and experimentation. Similarly, ideas for service delivery, arising from economic necessity, may offer the potential for widespread utilization.

What are the lessons to be learnt? Of course, wherever possible, planning for services ought to be done on the basis of sound data and an understanding of the socioeconomic influences behind those data, but where these are not available, a sensible pragmatic response has to be made incorporating the flexibility to develop in the light of new knowledge or later changes in practice.

We need to develop services appropriate to the geography of our area. As described by Mike Barnes, regional centres in urban areas can provide a focus for education, training and research. But the problems consequent on brain injury are not only immediate but also persistent and delayed. The regional unit can deal with early severe problems but perhaps should not be managing these later problems, both on geographical grounds or with regard to the potential number of clients involved. The regional centre, he argues, cannot be all things to all people and should certainly not substitute for the development of good quality, local rehabilitation services but rather complement them.

In the rural environment, locality-based, interdisciplinary teams as described by Chris Evans offer a useful model. What, though, of the peripatetic, physiotherapy service offered by Miroslav Palát? Could such a service, with its emphasis on family involvement, also play a key role in a comprehensive rural service? Palát, who developed the model, works in an urban area, where therapist travelling could be kept to a minimum. But patients in rural communities have great difficulty in travelling and community physiotherapists, given training in the needs of brain-injured patients, could surely deliver services (particularly in a monitoring and teaching as opposed to a 'hands-on' role) to rural patients.

The question of how far a specific intervention is generally applicable is an important one. Ina Berg and colleagues argue that specific approaches to the rehabilitation of memory problems, such as the use of mnemonics or a peg-word system, are not generally applied either by patients or, for that matter, by non-brain-injured controls. They, therefore, asked their patients to adopt strategies when assimilating or recalling information. But they confined their use of such strategies to patients who were without significant intellectual, aphasic, apraxic, agnosic or personality disturbances and only selected patients who were at least 9 months post-injury. We ask whether their approach could be applied more widely – to more severely affected patients, for example? Their observation that neurological factors and age did not affect favourable outcome seems to indicate this.

Fasotti and Kovács also approached the problem of lack of generalization of newly acquired skills by asking their patients to develop strategies, this time to circumvent slow information processing and its associated attentional problems. Their strategies, which were mainly aimed at reducing time-pressure during complex tasks, may also be applicable to a wider population than initially anticipated. However, as they point out, a behaviourist approach to learning certain tasks may be just as effective and may, perhaps, be more efficient when a task is to be carried out repeatedly and in the same manner each time. This approach has, for example, been used to enable a very severely amnesic patient to return to her closely structured job. Perhaps the next stage is to clarify which tasks are sufficiently routine to be taught using a behaviourist approach and which skills require generalizability and are, therefore, more appropriately learnt strategically. Indeed, perhaps patients need to be taught to ask themselves 'Will I carry out this task in exactly the same way each time or will I need to apply my newly acquired skill in several different situations?'

Ann Goodman-Smith's account of a behavioural approach to the management of severe emotional disturbance following brain injury is, in a sense, at the other extreme. Although some have criticized this approach as too specific, effective only within the confines of a behaviourist unit where all staff are aware of the goal and methods, one has to remember that she has used it with very severely impaired patients. It is also worth noting that units such as hers tend to take those few patients who have already tried many other approaches and failed. In such people, their subsequent lives are likely to follow a simple, regular structure. It may be hard for relatives to have to consider with the patient what is appropriate behaviour anew at every mealtime. Instead, it may be easier for the patient to be taught standard codes of behaviour at meals.

The lesson for relatives and carers from the behaviourist approach – that consistency is all-important – is relevant not just to behavioural treatments but to all forms of rehabilitation. Inconsistency not only hinders learning but also shakes confidence, particularly in the brain-injured person, recovering from coma, who may then feel disorientated and unsure of the nature of what is happening around him. In Vera Neumann's chapter the point is made that there has to be a consistency of aims and, preferably, of approaches from the professionals of varied backgrounds who can and should be enlisted to work in brain-injury rehabilitation teams. Each professional should be signed up to the agreed rehabilitation goals and aware of how his/her colleagues will be working towards these goals reflecting the value of the transdisciplinary team, as advocated by Finset [1].

Borrowing ideas from other areas is, one suspects, one method by which brain injury rehabilitation will develop. Consider, for example, the assessment process described by Agnes Sheil and her colleagues in Chapter 19. These authors point out the similarity to Portage techniques, which were initially developed for use in the field of developmental delay in children and which they are developing for use in brain injury management.

Debora Prichard and Eric Bérard have widened their approach to incorporate drama techniques in their workshops. Like Janet Cockburn and Jacqueline Wood, their concern was to make workshops resemble real life more closely and make them more relevant. This approach is refreshing. We should not be hidebound by rules about who, or what skills, should be in the rehabilitation team. There are often many possible solutions to a problem and many potential sources of help.

Janet Cockburn and her co-author also discuss the inappropriateness of measuring the responses to rehabilitation programmes by using measures developed to record impairments (not handicaps), which have been developed in other conditions, particularly stroke. These measures may be irrelevant for two reasons – firstly because the impairments are not the same in the two conditions, and secondly because the impairment cannot necessarily be expected to change in the course of rehabilitation, so that measurement must be of what can and should change. Thus, aphasia may not improve in a particular patient, but communication may, even to such an extent that the patient can return to work. At this stage the **handicap** has been reduced, not the impairment.

Handicap is, in part, determined by a patient's own goals and, indeed, individual satisfaction with treatment will depend on setting goals which are realistic, achievable and relevant. It is encouraging to see that the contributors to this book have veered away from the traditional approach to rehabilitation, where the goals (usually independence in mobility and self care) are set by the rehabilitation team, towards goals which patients have set and which are culturally relevant. There is likely to be less apathy attached to reaching these than, say, more traditional ones such as householding skills, which are not perceived by many young male patients as their goals.

Ina Berg and colleagues allowed their patients to define the memory problems which troubled them most, and Prichard and Bérard encouraged their groups to set their own tasks. It is also worth noting that management by case managers, who see themselves as patient advocates, and the increasing strength of Disability Rights Groups, particularly across Northern Europe and the United States of America, make goal-setting by institutions politically untenable.

What do case managers need to know? What training should they have? The community occupational therapy project carried out in Leeds (Chapter 6) describes how these occupational therapists, whose skills were previously not fully utilized as they were largely concerned with assessment of clients for stairlifts, rails and bathing equipment, welcomed training to screen for need in head-injured persons returning to the community. They were able to bring considerable help to patients and families, although their training in head injury was neither costly nor lengthy. Subsequently a small peripatetic team, including not only an occupational therapist but two other professionals, has provided a focus for the solution of such problems. Further research may be required to determine what the skill mix of such a resource should be, but, in essence, benefit probably accrues when fragmentation of skills and information are replaced by a focused, knowledgeable team or group of professionals with a high profile so that referral to them is easy and access equitable. It is likely that the small team has a greater range of assessment and therapeutic skills than a lone case manager, although this statement has yet to be proved.

Michael Oddy describes how he has helped relatives to come to terms with changed personality, the process being mainly one of information giving. Hopefully, this and the provision of available community help will prevent head-injured people from being inappropriately placed in long-term institutional care. However, as Oddy points out, there is no simple answer for all situations. Some relatives must actually be helped towards making a decision of opting not to be carers. Some head-injured people will flourish in institutions: not all are large and lacking in stimulation and friendship. The best are self-sufficient communities offering sheltered work and a sense of purpose and belonging [2]. While, in Britain at least, the emphasis is on placing all in the 'community', this can be a lonely place – sitting at home, by oneself, for years on end, perhaps occasionally attending a day centre for the very elderly, may not represent anything more than existing.

Given all our efforts to establish an appropriate service structure and to offer the best treatment, it is imperative that we measure what we do. We have to demonstrate that the new service structure is better than the old. To do this we must have valid, reliable and sensitive measures.

The WHO classification (ICIDH) [3] has made a major contribution by helping us to think analytically: it crosses language barriers. In our own thinking and in our proposed measures we have to be clear about the differences between impairment, disability and handicap. Many of our traditional outcome measures are of impairment or disability, when in reality the challenge is in the area of handicap and in the impact of the injury as perceived by an individual and society. The adjustments that have to be made lie within the fields not only of physical independence but of the fruitful occupation of time and economic self-sufficiency.

Much work still needs to be done to develop measures which allow assignment to the various ICIDH categories, particularly those concerned with occupation, economic independence and social integration. But we should not be constrained by the limitations of our current standardized measurements. Shiel and Horn's work reminds us that changes in independence, for instance, may be occurring which do not produce an improvement measurable on any standard scale, but which can be accurately recorded by documenting functional behaviour in a systematic way. Such a system allows us to record change, even when this is too small or large for standard scales. This, in turn, can guide therapy appropriately.

We progress by the sharing of ideas and the continual questioning of existing methods. In brain injury the objective is simple – though the problem is inordinately complex. We strive to improve the lives of those who have sustained traumatic brain injury. We hope this book has made a contribution towards that end.

REFERENCES

1. Finset A. Subacute brain injury rehabilitation: a program description and a study of staff program evaluation. *Scandinavian Journal of Rehabilitation Medicine* 1992; **26**(Suppl): 25–33.
2. Hunter R, MacAlpine I. *Psychiatry for the Poor*. Folkestone: William Dawson & Sons, 1974.
3. World Health Organization. *The International Classification of Impairments, Disablities and Handicaps*. Geneva: World Health Organization, 1980.

Index

Page numbers in **bold** refer to figures and page numbers in *italics* to tables.